*un*scripted

the unpredictable moments
that make life EXTRAORDINARY

ERNIE JOHNSON JR.

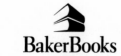

BakerBooks
a division of Baker Publishing Group
Grand Rapids, Michigan

Published by Baker Books
a division of Baker Publishing Group
PO Box 6287, Grand Rapids, MI 49516-6287
www.bakerbooks.com

Paper edition published 2018
ISBN 978-0-8010-9373-9

Printed in the United States of America

The Library of Congress has cataloged the original edition as follows:
Names: Johnson, Ernie, 1956– author.
Title: Unscripted : the unpredictable moments that make life extraordinary / Ernie Johnson Jr.
Description: Grand Rapids : Baker Books, 2017. | Includes bibliographical references and index.
Identifiers: LCCN 2016052074 | ISBN 9780801074103 (pbk. : alk. paper)
Subjects: LCSH: Johnson, Ernie, 1956– | Johnson, Ernie, 1956– —Religion. | Sportscasters—United States—Biography. | Cancer—Patients—United States—Biography. | Parents of children with disabilities—United States—Biography.
Classification: LCC GV742.42.J65 A3 2017 | DDC 070.4/49796092 [B]—dc23
LC record available at https://lccn.loc.gov/2016052074

In keeping with biblical principles of creation stewardship, Baker Publishing Group advocates the responsible use of our natural resources. As a member of the Green Press Initiative, our company uses recycled paper when possible. The text paper of this book is composed in part of post-consumer waste.

18 19 20 21 22 23 24   7 6 5 4 3 2 1

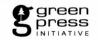

"Ernie has been an example to me of how to balance the demands of work with those of your family. He has remained humble in an industry that doesn't reward humility. Most importantly, he has truly put the Lord first in his life. In *Unscripted*, you will enjoy some wonderful sports stories, but more than that, you will learn some invaluable life lessons."

Tony Dungy, bestselling author of *Quiet Strength* and *Uncommon*

"Most people know Ernie as a guy who has been broadcasting for four decades. I am one of the lucky ones who know him as an extraordinary man and a friend. *Unscripted* gives everyone a glimpse of a life well lived and a man with tremendous perspective, humor, and class."

Cal Ripken, Hall of Famer and baseball's all-time "Iron Man"

"If you know Ernie only as the man behind the microphone, you are in for a treat. Here is Ernie Johnson, a great man of our time."

Max Lucado, pastor and bestselling author

"Ernie quite simply is one of the best people on the planet."

Charles Barkley, *Inside the NBA* on TNT

"I have known Ernie for almost two decades, and he has had tremendous influence in my life and in my thinking. His is a faith that is simple but very deep. And you see it lived out in every relationship in his life. When he speaks, you'd be wise to listen. I know I do."

Jeff Foxworthy, comedian and author

"Just thinking of Ernie Johnson puts a smile on my face. For as long as I've been blessed to know him, he has been a source of inspiration. I admire his devotion to his beautiful family and talented colleagues. *Unscripted* best describes this uplifting book . . . and Ernie himself. Despite the many challenges my friend has faced, you'll be in awe of his faith and desire to be of service to others."

Robin Roberts, *Good Morning America* on ABC

"I promise you will be moved and inspired by Ernie's story. This book could quite possibly transform your attitude as well as your heart toward all of life. As I read it, I found myself wanting to be a better man. *Unscripted* is a must-read, and I know you will be as captivated as I was when you read it."

From the foreword by **John Smoltz**,
Hall of Fame pitcher, Atlanta Braves

"Ernie Johnson is an extraordinary man. He has lived an amazing life, absent of ego but bountiful with experiences that are soulful and warmhearted. Stories about family, faith, and fellowship. He said one of the driving forces behind this book was to make his father proud. He has done that a thousandfold . . . and has shined a light on both our industry and goodness in the world. EJ has introduced me to an important new phrase, a "blackberry moment." If you are not inspired after reading this, you are not human. *Unscripted* is unforgettable!"

Jim Nantz, CBS Sports

"Great to see Ernie putting his thoughts to paper with *Unscripted*. His life and insight are unparalleled, and it's time the world sees what we see daily."

Kenny "The Jet" Smith, *Inside the NBA* on TNT

"Unscripted has it all . . . sports, high-wire pressure, behind-the-scenes-secrets, winning and losing, pain and hope, life and death, family and faith, and what matters most. Ernie blends this into a fabulous story that will for sure grip your imagination and just might change your life. Turns out there may be a script after all."

John Ortberg, senior pastor of Menlo Church;
author of *All the Places to Go*

"I have known Ernie since I was starting off in the business over thirty years ago, and have come to admire and appreciate him as a member of the sportscasting "family" . . . and as a family man. With *Unscripted*, Ernie captures the challenges of building a singular career in the public eye, while devoting himself to his job as a spouse and parent. His snapshots of pride, fear, joy, sadness, compassion, and hope will resonate with readers, no matter their industry or family structure. "Unscripted" moments are the stuff of our lives, and Ernie offers a personal and lasting triumph in this regard, far from the bright lights of sports television."

Hannah Storm, *SportsCenter* on ESPN;
award-winning producer and director

"One of the most genuine voices I've encountered. Ernie's contribution to sports and media is noteworthy, but his investment into the lives of others is a story all its own."

Lecrae, Grammy Award–winning rapper
and songwriter

"Every time I've had the privilege of hearing my friend Ernie share parts of his story, I've been encouraged, blessed, undone, challenged, and amazed by the remarkable faith and trust that has marked his life and his journey. I'm so thankful that he has written his story and given us this incredible gift of *Unscripted* so many others can be inspired the way I've been by knowing this great man, friend, husband, and dad."

Steven Curtis Chapman, five-time Grammy Award winner

"Ernie Johnson is one of the finest men I've ever known. Not just in sports. Not just in sports television. He's one of the best men I've ever met. Period. I treasure his friendship."

Verne Lundquist, sportscaster for CBS Sports

"Ernie Johnson is a living example of the truth "It's not what happens to you but how you handle what happens to you." He is exceptional and inspirational, a person I highly respect."

James Brown, CBS Sports & News

"Whether a sports fan or not, you will find this book to be a complete delight. I will never look at blackberries the same. Read it!"

William Paul Young, bestselling author of *The Shack*,
Cross Roads, and *Eve*

"Ernie Johnson has been sportscasting exciting games for decades, and yet no moment about barreling into home plate, sinking the putt, or hitting the game-winning shot compares to the true story of his family. We love Ernie and his family for the same reason we love sports; something about us resonates with the broken hero just trying to find home. This book has more glory in it than a thousand World Series, and the characters are no less enticing."

Donald Miller, bestselling author of *Blue Like Jazz*

"*Unscripted* is how all of our lives begin. Some choose to do more with their lives. Ernie Johnson is one of those people. Although Ernie and I are about the same age, I always feel as though he is the older brother I never had. Ernie makes everyone feel related or connected in his own gracious way. When we are working together for Turner Sports, he will always pay homage to his father by saying "We are zipping right along here in the 6th inning," and I will turn to him and we exchange a quiet nod. That phrase will be etched in my brain forever. Simply every minute I spend with Ernie makes me aspire to be a better man."

Ronnie Darling Jr., Turner Sports

"Ernie Johnson is one of the most talented and versatile broadcast journalists in our business. He's knowledgeable, personable, and generous with his time. I'm so happy to finally see his journey to the top recorded in *Unscripted*."

William C. Rhoden, author of *Forty Million Dollar Slaves: The Rise, Fall and Redemption of the Black Athlete*

"After having the honor of personally knowing Ernie for many years now, and seeing his faith and heart lived out in his words and deeds, it is such a pleasure to read more stories and insights into the life of my good friend EJ!"

Mac Powell, lead vocalist and songwriter for Grammy Award–winning band Third Day

In honor of my father, Ernie Johnson Sr.
In admiration of my mother, Lois
In gratitude to my sisters, Dawn and Chris
In love with my wife, Cheryl, and our amazing kids,
Eric, Maggie, Michael, Carmen, Allison, and Ashley

CONTENTS

FOREWORD

I HAVE ENCOUNTERED all kinds of people in the sport of baseball as well as outside of sports, and hands down Ernie Johnson Jr. is one of my favorites in the world. Ernie and I go way back—back to the days when his father called Braves games, games where I was on the mound doing my best to throw out the next batter.

As a pitcher you have the luxury of working five days and then listening or watching games four days. I would catch games on TV from the clubhouse while charting games and listening to the Braves' broadcasters. Ernie Johnson Sr.'s voice was one I came to rely on and cherish. In addition, the players travel with the broadcasters, so we were all one big family.

I have gotten to know Ernie Jr. as well and saw the bond that he and his dad shared. These days, we hang out once a week, if our schedules allow, in a Bible study with some other guys. (You'll read about us in these pages.) So when I say I know Ernie, I say that not only because the same sport employed us but because we have spent quite a bit of personal time with each other. I've gotten to know his heart, and what a heart it is.

We used to have more time together, Ernie Jr. and I. After retiring, I got to work alongside him calling games for TBS. I will never forget those times we had, traveling together and witnessing some historic plays. It was then that I witnessed his struggles and family moments that all of us have to deal with. The way he handled these struggles—struggles that stretched his faith and patience beyond what most of us could handle—will forever be stitched in my mind. You're a giant, Ernie.

Now I am going to confess something I probably shouldn't. Truth is, I have started and failed to finish many books. But I finished *Unscripted* in three days, which in and of itself is a major thing for me. But more importantly, it's a testament to this: Never will I find a finer man than Ernie Johnson, whose profound humility and love for God and his family are so evident here. Ernie is not perfect and has not done everything right in his life, but he has a deep desire to live a purposeful life that honors God.

I promise you will be moved and inspired by his story. This book could quite possibly transform your attitude as well as your heart toward all of life. As I read it, I found myself wanting to be a better man. *Unscripted* is a must-read, and I know you will be as captivated as I was when you read it.

John Smoltz, Atlanta Braves pitcher, Hall of Fame 2015

INTRODUCTION

IF YOU INCLUDE THE VERY FIRST TIME I sat behind a microphone as a twenty-year-old, sweaty-palmed junior at WUOG, the University of Georgia's student radio station, I have been broadcasting for forty years now. I've made my living on television for the last thirty-eight, most of those as a sportscaster, and yet there is no guarantee you know who I am.

Maybe you're not a sports fan, or perhaps you've made a conscious effort to keep your TV viewing to a minimum. I have no problem with that; in fact, my wife, Cheryl, fits that description on both counts, especially the "not a sports fan" part of that equation. In the pages that follow, you'll get to know Cheryl very well, and I am certain you will find her as enchanting as I did when I met her thirty-seven years ago.

So all of that being said, let me introduce myself. I am Ernie Johnson Jr. Those of you who already know me from my work on the Turner networks, TNT and TBS, will probably refer to me as the guy who hosts the show *Inside the NBA*, which features NBA Hall of Famers Charles Barkley and Shaquille O'Neal and two-time NBA champion Kenny Smith, or as the guy who calls Major League Baseball with another Hall of Famer, Cal Ripken, and all-star pitcher Ron Darling. Still, while my appearances on television perhaps gave you a clear idea of what I *do*, they did not necessarily tell you who I *am*.

That changed dramatically in the spring of 2015.

It is quite rare in my business for one network to air a feature on a personality from a competing network, but that is exactly what happened in 2015. Jeremy Schaap, an award-winning journalist for ESPN, approached me about producing a profile of my family. He was aware that my wife, Cheryl, and I are the parents of six children, four of whom are adopted, three of whom have special-needs, and one of whom has a fatal disease (muscular dystrophy). Jeremy knew of my past battle with cancer and about the bond I shared with my late father, another longtime broadcaster, Ernie Johnson Sr.

Jeremy wanted to tell my story on the network's *E:60* news-magazine show. My wife and I were hesitant at first to allow television cameras that kind of access into what had always been a very private part of our lives. But then we thought about the possible benefits. What if this feature struck a chord with parents who were considering adoption or were going through the daily rigors of caring for a special-needs child? What if it encouraged a man or a woman faced with the reality of chemotherapy? Or what if it helped to strengthen or repair the relationship between a father and a son?

We agreed to allow Jeremy and his producer, Dan Lindberg, to have at it. What they produced—a twenty-five-minute feature titled *My Story: Ernie Johnson Jr.*—did all of the things

Cheryl and I prayed it would. The response was staggering and humbling, and more than a year later, as the program has re-aired and been distributed online, I continue to hear from fathers and sons and cancer patients and adoptive parents and moms and dads with special-needs kids who were impacted in some way by the heartfelt presentation Jeremy and Dan produced. We are eternally grateful.

And so now I have done something I have long thought about doing, even before that *E:60* piece was ever conceived. I have written a book—the one you're holding. I call it *Unscripted* not only because it is the perfect description of the show I am blessed to work on with Charles, Shaq, and Kenny but also because my life away from the TV cameras has been one unscripted, unforeseen, unforgettable moment after another.

My wish is not that you regard our family in some glorified, elevated way. Far from it. My wish is that this book will speak to you on some level right where you live in the area of parenting or faith or heartbreak or triumph.

And my wish is that this book will honor my father.

And my heavenly Father.

Here's to embracing the unscripted.

Enjoy.

1

Blackberries

IT WAS A FASTBALL, about belt high. I say "fast" meaning it was a straight pitch, not a curveball or a slider. Dads whose sons were in a league of eight- and soon-to-be nine-year-olds in the mid-1960s didn't let their sons throw breaking stuff.

Anyway, I had a good look at this belt-high fastball from my position at shortstop in a game that we, the Vees (don't ask, I don't know), were leading by a couple runs. That lead was in jeopardy because this belt-high fastball, which I had such a good look at, was lined over my head before I had a chance to take my glove off my knee. It bounced once in left center field and cleared the chain-link fence, which no player in our league had ever cleared on a hop, much less on the fly, so this ground-rule double was pretty impressive in my book.

The hit scored the runners from second and third and tied the game. This necessitated a meeting on the mound so our coach could tell us, the infielders, what we should do if the next ball was hit to us now that the go-ahead runner stood at second, still grinning about his display of eight-year-old power. The coach had his say. We nodded as if we understood the defensive strategy he had outlined, though I'm pretty sure our first baseman was thinking more about how good a snow cone would taste when this game was over. So was I. It may have been an early Saturday morning, but it was Georgia, and it was hot. It was "try not to think about snow cones in the middle of the game" hot. And so we, the Vees (look, maybe the league was just using the alphabet to name teams; I don't know, so stop asking), trotted back to our positions, and that's when this story, for me, became worth telling.

You see, before another pitch could be thrown, we had to find two of our outfielders. When that belt-high fastball had been sent screaming, or at least speaking in more than an indoor voice, over my head and into the gap, our left fielder and center fielder had converged and had had the best seats in the house to watch the ball hit the grass and disappear into the trees and bushes and underbrush that adorned this part of the ballpark where no ball had ever gone before. And during our meeting of the minds on the mound, they apparently had taken it upon themselves to climb the chain-link fence and retrieve the "Official League" baseball. This was not necessary because, while the league may have been strapped when it came to naming its teams, I am certain the umpiring crew was equipped with more than one baseball for a game of this magnitude. Perhaps they had wanted to find that ball and award it to the peewee power hitter, who was now flexing his biceps at second base while waiting for play to resume. Whatever their motives, the search was under way, and the rest of us Vees (don't even . . .) sprinted toward the fence to provide encouragement, or point to where we thought the ball had gone, or simply ask, "Why are you on that side of the fence?"

As it turns out, this was not a search that would require a compass or bloodhounds or even twenty-twenty eyesight. The ball had come to rest in plain sight about ten feet past the fence. Our two missing outfielders had seen it. But they had also discovered a blackberry bramble, and it was filled with a mother lode of ripe and apparently delicious blackberries. While the infielders were getting chapter and verse from the coach on what to do if the ball was hit in our direction, our left fielder and center fielder were stretching their skinny arms through the bramble, deftly avoiding the menacing thorns, rejoicing in their discovery, and testifying to another reason this game is indeed our national pastime.

I'll be the first to admit this may not be a thigh-slapping, gut-busting story. It is unlikely anyone who hears it will immediately jump on their Twitter account and give it an LOL. It probably falls more into the "Oh, isn't that amusing?" category. But a game that features a blackberry delay struck a chord with my dad. And oh, by the way, I have no memory of how the rest of that game turned out. From that point on, it simply became "the blackberry moment."

It would be years before that story became, for me, more than the tale of a Little League game delayed. We would tell and retell that story in our family and laugh each time as if we'd just gotten back from the ballpark. My father was a major league pitcher in the 1950s, most notably as a reliever for those great Milwaukee Braves teams, and he delighted in the innocence of that story. As he transitioned from the playing field to the broadcast booth, as the Braves moved from Milwaukee to Atlanta, he was a regular on the banquet and luncheon circuits. If you were a member of the Kiwanis Club, the Optimist Club, the Jaycees, the Rotary Club, or the Salvation Army, you heard Ernie Johnson Sr. deliver a speech.

I loved to tag along. I loved to hear again what the members of those clubs were hearing for the first time. What it was like to play alongside the likes of Hank Aaron and Eddie Mathews and Warren Spahn and Lou Burdette. What it was like to pitch to Stan Musial and Ted Williams and Jackie Robinson. And what was even better than hearing my dad tell those stories was hearing and seeing the reaction. Belly laughs . . . palms hitting tables, making silverware clink against plates and drinking glasses . . . middle-aged men trying to catch their breath before the old right-hander uncorked another gem from the memory bank.

Every once in a while he'd throw this one in: "And then there was that morning when little Ernie, and he's seated right down here in front, was playing a peewee game over at Murphey Candler Park. . . ." And the story of the blackberry moment would be told by the greatest storyteller I ever knew.

In many ways that story has become central to my perspective on you name it: work, relaxation—shoot, life. It's a kind of parable about not being afraid to step away from the game (translated the job, the meeting, the conference call, the list of emails, the seemingly pressing matter at hand) to appreciate the unexpected, unscripted moments. When I stop to think about it, it's always the blackberry moments that stand out when I think about the wide variety of sports I've had the chance to be a part of in the winding course of my career.

In 1998, I was doing track and field play-by-play at the World Cup finals in Johannesburg, South Africa. Know what I remember most about that trip? Not the 100- and 200-meter golds won by Marion Jones, remarkable as they were. No, it was a visit to Soweto a day or two before the runners ran, the pole-vaulters vaulted, the high jumpers jumped, and the steeplechasers did whatever steeplechasers do. I'd heard about Soweto. It was a focal point in the fight against apartheid. It was there in June of 1976 that thousands of high school students staged a protest march—the Soweto Uprising—that turned deadly as South African authorities opened fire.

Now, twenty-two years later, I was riding in a van with a producer and a video crew following a busload of US athletes to the township where a new sports center for kids had been built. I looked out the window of the van at the rows upon rows of what were basically tiny huts with tin roofs, thinking at times it appeared a neighborhood had been built on a landfill. And I saw this brand-new facility and this sea of kids and parents waiting outside for this busload of athletes to arrive. And I remember the smiles. I still have photos of that day on the shelves of my home office, and every time I look at those snapshots I see something new and the feeling of that day returns and I feel lucky. USA Track and Field gave us T-shirts to give out to the kids, and I have pictures of tiny kids wearing extra-large T-shirts that nearly touched the ground. There's a picture of me reaching to shake hands with a group of kids, and they're laughing, and so are the moms and a grandmother. There are looks on faces that say, "Who's this guy with the receding hairline and the plastic credential hanging around his neck?" or "What's with this hand extended . . . Do you want me to slap it or shake it?" Oh, that day was marvelous. And I remember, as we drove back to our Johannesburg hotel that evening, we saw the sun setting in our rearview mirror so brilliantly that we had to pull over so we could take pictures. The Creator had his paintbrush out again, and it was a spectacular finish to an unforgettable day.

I'll tell you the truth. I had to look up on the internet the highlights of that 1998 track meet, but I will never forget those Soweto images or that sunset. That's what unscripted blackberry moments do. I think God has placed blackberry brambles along the paths we walk every day. We just need the eyes to see them, the ears to hear them, and the hearts to detect them. All that stands in the way is the busyness of life. We're all so focused on sticking to the script from one day to the next, one meeting to the next, one sales call to the next, that we blow right by the unscripted moments that can profoundly impact not just our lives but also the lives of those with whom we share the planet, the workplace, or a home. If there's one thing life has taught me, it's not to *fear* the unscripted but to *embrace* it.

On August 16, 2011, the story of the blackberry moment at that Little League park and all it has meant occupied my every thought. Soon it would come spilling from my own lips as I delivered my father's eulogy.

2

Dad

MY FATHER HAD HAIRY EARS. Check that. He had really, really hairy ears. He had "Hey, what are you doin' wearin' earmuffs in the middle of summer?" hairy ears. When I would see an infomercial on late-night TV extolling the virtues of a state-of-the-art trimmer that could remove unsightly nose and ear hairs, I would dismiss its claims outright because the manufacturers had obviously never tried that thing out on Ernest Thorwald Johnson Sr. I would go so far as to say that the folks who make Weed Eaters would have been at least a bit intimidated by the sight. I wondered sometimes when he asked me to repeat something I'd said to him if my words hadn't gotten tangled up in that underbrush and never reached his eardrums. So where's this going? you ask. I'm getting there.

In the last month or so of my father's days, before congestive heart failure brought the curtain down on what was a George Bailey–style wonderful life, he lived for a short time in an Atlanta rehabilitation center. Ernie Senior, or Big Guy, as we called him around the house, or Poppy, as the grand-children called him, or the right-hander, as I called him when we worked Atlanta Braves telecasts in the mid-1990s, was six foot four, a great athlete whose talents had taken him to the major leagues as a pitcher for the Milwaukee Braves and the Baltimore Orioles in the 1950s. Now at the age of eighty-seven, he was struggling. Strength, energy, balance—they were all leaving him. And so was his memory. His mind was playing tricks on him. The early stages of Alzheimer's had become more and more evident. I think that was the most difficult part of his illness for our family to witness. My dad's loss of access to the vault of memories he'd accumulated was heartbreaking.

One afternoon in the rehab center's living room/sunroom/visiting area for families, I finally did something with my dad I had never done before. I trimmed those hairy ears. The trimmer, with a fresh, right-outta-the-package battery, hummed as I turned it on. With the trimmer inches from my dad's left ear, I began to wonder if there was any fine print in the instruction manual detailing what to do if the device became jammed or entangled in hair too dense for this model to handle. But I forged ahead, and with great success, I might add. In fact, the left ear was going so well that I thought I'd have to ask the janitorial staff if they had a broom and a dustpan I could borrow. Dad and I laughed about what had to be an interesting if not comedic scene for others in the room, and as I moved to the other side, I couldn't help but wonder what was going on *between* my dad's ears. What if he had lost the ability to remember things the rest of us thought we'd never forget?

Did he remember growing up in Vermont? That's where he was born to Swedish parents, Thorwald and Ingeborg. That's where he spent time ski jumping and ice-skating and becoming a star baseball, basketball, and football player at Brattleboro High School. Did he remember the first time he laid eyes on that cheerleader, Lois Denhard, who would become his wife of sixty-three years? How about his World War II tour of duty with the United States Marine Corps in the Pacific? The unbreakable bonds he forged with his brothers in arms there, with whom he would remain in contact for years to come until slowly their numbers dwindled?

How well did he remember, I wondered, that glorious 1957 World Series in which he was a relief pitcher for the Milwaukee Braves, playing alongside legends such as Hank Aaron, Eddie Mathews, Warren Spahn, and Lou Burdette? Did he remember being my seventh-grade basketball coach at St. Jude's outside Atlanta—benching me for not playing tough enough in one game and later celebrating with me when my two free throws in the closing seconds gave us the championship? (In all honesty, the other team, Westminster, had fouled me intentionally, knowing there was no way the scrawny kid would hit two pressure free throws. Had I been coaching Westminster I would have done the same thing.)

Did he recall how my two older sisters, Dawn and Chris, and I would sneak up behind him while he sat in his easy chair in the den and play with his hair? He had a special way of spreading it around so that his head was pretty much covered. It wasn't a comb-over as much as it was a "swirl" on top of his head, so if you caught him unaware, you could actually scoop up his hair and extend it straight up a good seven or eight inches. It was a wondrous sight. He would feign annoyance—"C'mon, you guys"—but it was always said with a laugh, so we never stopped doing it.

Did he remember all the piano recitals Dawn and Chris had participated in and those early morning or late afternoon horseback rides with Chris? How about those Christmas Day games of H-O-R-S-E on the driveway basketball "court" when we spent as much time retrieving the ball from the woods as we did shooting it? Everybody in the family played, which led to some marathon games, but there were so many laughs that nobody cared. How about that one round of golf we played at Augusta National? If you're not into golf, Augusta National is the site of the Masters Tournament every year and is basically the Sistine Chapel of the sport. Did he remember how lucky we were to be playing golf on December 10, 1998, on a seventy-degree day, putting on the same greens that the greats of the game had putted on and walking the same fairways? (Okay, for those of you who are wondering, he beat me by a couple strokes, and we both broke a hundred.) So many blackberry moments in a life that spanned nearly ninety years.

As I finished with his right ear and the trimmer's smooth hum was replaced by a labored groan, I stepped back not only to admire my handiwork but also to gaze at the man I had always wanted to be.

Back in the day (that's athletespeak for "a long time ago"), it wasn't always enough for a Major League Baseball player just to be a Major League Baseball player. Salaries weren't that great "back in the day," so Dad had a job during the off-season selling insurance for Northwestern Mutual. I had always wanted to be a baseball player like him, but in the winter, I had wanted to wear a long-sleeved white business shirt just like he would wear to work. My exact wish, my mom says, went like this: "I want to wear a white shirt where the sleeves go down like an insurance man." When his playing days were through, Dad did not make a career of the insurance business. Baseball was in Big Guy's blood. The Milwaukee Braves made him their public relations director and later a member of the broadcast team after the franchise moved to Atlanta in the mid-1960s. And that is when my education truly began. It was then my father became the greatest influence in my life.

Growing up as the son of a broadcaster certainly had its perks, no doubt about it. Not many kids can tag along with their dad to the ballpark, hang out around the batting cage, and listen to Hank Aaron ask you how your Little League team is doing. I also got the chance simply to watch Dad work. I don't think he realized it at the time, but he was teaching me without ever actually trying. I watched his meticulous game preparation. He was always among the first to arrive at the park and never rushed through the pregame work that needed to be done. I listened to him interview players and managers and then sat in the radio booth during the game, watching and listening as he called the game. To this day, baseball fans who used to listen to him tell me, "I got to talk to your dad once, and he sounded just the same in person as he did on the radio." No surprise there. Dad's mantra was "Be yourself." He never put on airs, never tried to create some persona. He was simply "good old Ernie" to viewers and listeners.

But his greatest teaching didn't come on the field or in the booth. It came on the walk from the field to the press box. Fans who came early to watch batting practice would without fail beckon to my dad from fifty yards away. "Hey, Ernie!" would come the call from an unknown voice. After my father turned and made his way through the blue wooden seats of Atlanta–Fulton County Stadium to come face-to-face with the owner of that unfamiliar voice, he would hear a familiar tale. "Man, we listen to you all the time. We came up here from Macon and just wanted to say hi." And my dad would spend time with these strangers as if they were lifelong friends.

I have volumes of mental notes from meetings like that. My dad wasn't lecturing me about respect; he was demonstrating it. He wasn't preaching to me about humility; he was modeling it. During one particular broadcast, shortly after Skip Caray and Pete Van Wieren were hired to be Dad's partners, Skip came out of a commercial break and said, "We head to the top of the fourth, and to call it for you, here again is the voice of the Braves, Ernie Johnson." Dad did the play-by-play for that half inning and then during the next set of commercials turned to Skip and said, "Hey, if it's all right with you, Skip, you don't need to introduce me that way. You and me and Pete—we're all the voice of the Braves." That's just the way he was. Just being himself—Big Guy.

Those lessons learned at the ballpark during my teenage years would be a guiding light as my professional career began. The baseball player thing never quite panned out for me. I walked on as a freshman at the University of Georgia and was told to walk off as a sophomore. There aren't many roster spots available for guys who are good with the glove but can't hit their weight. That was me. So having spent so much time watching my dad work in broadcasting, I decided to try it too. From a radio station in Athens, Georgia, to

TV jobs in Macon and Spartanburg, South Carolina, and Atlanta, and then eventually to Turner Broadcasting, I have heard my father's voice.

- "Be yourself."
- "Don't think you're special because of the job you have."
- "Never think you're bigger than the game."
- "Treat everyone with respect."
- "Be loyal."
- "Once you've done your best, to heck with it."
- "Take the high road."

I need to spend a moment or two on that last one because to this day it remains very much a guidepost, especially in my professional career. No matter what line of work you're in, there will be times when you're criticized or when you feel a co-worker has done you wrong—maybe done something behind your back to elevate his or her value and at the same time diminish yours. Back in the 1970s, long before anybody thought of Twitter and its ability to deliver up-to-the-second opinions on everything from breaking news to celebrity gossip, there was fan mail. Grasp the concept. Actually write a letter, put it in an envelope, put a stamp on it, and then wonder if the intended recipient in fact received it and would have the inclination to respond. My dad got a ton of fan mail as an Atlanta Braves announcer and did his best to respond to all of it.

Sometimes I would sit in his office at the stadium hours before a game and read those letters from fans praising the quality of the Braves' broadcasts, telling my dad how much they enjoyed listening to him. His fan mail was predominantly positive, but some letters were, how should I put it, not so nice, or downright rude, and Dad would make it a point to bring those home and let us read them. As a teenager in those days, I was outraged when a fan attacked my father in writing.

"Dad, you've gotta write this guy back and let him have it. You can't let him get away with this stuff."

Dad would just laugh it off.

"You're never going to make everybody happy in this business, Ernst." He rarely called me Ernie when I was growing up. It was usually Tiger or Ernst, an abbreviated form of my given name, Ernest. "Just take the high road, Ernst. Never get into a pissin' fight with a skunk."

Dad would respond to the bad fan mail as well as the good, and often when he answered one of those mean-spirited letters, it would be with a postcard that featured a photo of the Braves' broadcast team. His handwritten reply would read, "Thanks for taking the time to write, and thanks for listening. Glad you're a Braves fan." I always wished I could be there to watch somebody who had unloaded on my father open that letter and realize that instead of having his fire returned in kind, he was dealing with a guy who lived on the high road. It was good teaching. Like every other on-air personality, I've taken more than my share of shots from viewers, especially in this social media age, and it always serves me well to remember my dad's words.

Now, while baseball was something to which my father devoted his professional life, I learned even more from him away from the ballpark. I watched my dad being a dad—making the time, when there wasn't much time to be had, to be with us. Even when baseball season had ended, as the

Braves' director of broadcasting, he still had to go to work, setting up the Braves' network of radio stations around the Southeast that would carry the team's broadcasts in the upcoming season. I think of the times he worked all day, drove a half hour or forty-five minutes home from downtown, and then turned right around and drove back downtown with me in the passenger seat so we could watch the Atlanta Hawks play basketball or the Atlanta Flames play hockey.

Now don't get me wrong—it wasn't all fun and games, and if you're a parent, you know what I mean. The man could lay down the law. Sure, I got some spankings, but what I remember more are things like the lecture he gave me when he found out that his son, altar boy in the making, had not bothered to try to learn the Latin liturgy required at the time. It ranks as one of the great dressing-downs ever administered by a parent to his child. I woke up the next morning reciting, *Kyrie Eleison* and *Et cum spiritu tuo* as if I'd been born and raised in Vatican City!

My father knew how to nurture a friendship with me while at the same time leaving absolutely no doubt about our assigned roles. I could be his golfing buddy one day, and then later that week he could be judge and jury. I remember how excited a friend and I were about the prospect of driving from Atlanta to North Carolina one weekend for an outdoor concert that featured one of my favorite bands—Emerson, Lake and Palmer. We had it all worked out, and my friend's parents had given their okay. Now all I needed was for mine to sign off on it. My mother wasn't thrilled with the idea. She conjured up visions of Woodstock, drugs, and motor-cycle gangs. She said my father would have the final say. He came home from the ballpark on Friday night as my friend and I waited, hoping we were just a matter of hours from hitting the road. Mom told him we were in the living room awaiting his verdict. As he started up the stairs to the bedroom, he poked his head into the living room and delivered a judgment that was controlled, remarkably swift, and left no room for rebuttal.

"I'm gonna be the horse's ass here, fellas. You're not going. Good night."

While there was no masking my disappointment, deep down I did have an appreciation, even in that moment, for the kind of father I had. I always knew where I stood. And I knew he loved me. But, man, that would have been a great concert.

When I got married in 1982, there was no question who my best man would be. It would be the guy who had encouraged, corrected, and inspired me for twenty-six years. My gift to him on that August morning was a pewter beer mug engraved with six words: "My Best Man. My Best Friend." And on another August morning twenty-nine years later, I stood at the lectern at St. Jude's Catholic Church and tried to get through the toughest thing I'll ever do with a microphone in front of me: eulogize my best friend. It was unscripted. I had jotted down a few notes as a road map of sorts for where I wanted to go. The blackberry story I've already described was the starting point, and the rest went as follows:

> In Paul's letter to the Galatians, chapter 5, verses 22 through 23, it says the fruits of the Spirit are love and joy, peace and patience, kindness, goodness, faithfulness, gentleness, and self-control. And my dad lived that. Paul was writing the letter to believers in Jesus Christ, and these are the trademarks,

the earmarks, of the Holy Spirit–led life. I can honestly say that my sisters, Chris and Dawn, and I thoroughly tested the outer reaches of the self-control and the gentleness. We tested the goodness and kindness and patience and peace. But never the faithfulness and never the love—never tested it.

Paul goes on in his second letter to Timothy, and at this point he knows his death is near. He says, "I have fought the good fight, I have finished the race, I have kept the faith. Now there is in store for me the crown of righteousness, which the Lord, the righteous Judge, will award to me on that day—and not only to me, but also to all who have longed for his appearing" [4:7–8].

I have no doubts where the right-hander is today. As my son Michael told me the other day . . . Michael has been zippin' around in a wheelchair, sitting there in the second row . . . He said, "Poppy is in heaven with God and Jesus and the angels." And he's right. And I'm sure he's heard the words, "Well done, good and faithful servant." And I'm sure he's hearing some stories that are even better than the ones you've heard today. And I'd like to add just a couple to them.

God has given us so many moments that blessed us and blessed those who seek them. I call those blackberries. And those blackberry moments, if we get too tied up in what we're doing in our jobs, in the game, in whatever it is, we miss them, and when we do, we're missing out on so much.

My life has been filled with them. Our family's been filled with them. There were some blackberries for my sister Chris. She said, "My dad was the perfect dad for a tomboy. He realized a fishing pole was just as good a fit as a Barbie doll for girls like me and taught me to fish when I was five years old. It was a hobby we shared for over fifty years. He let me take horseback riding lessons when I was twelve. We used to go riding in the fall when baseball season was over." That was spreading blackberries with a fishing pole and horseback riding. And my sister Dawn was all about the wintertime. My dad, having grown up in Vermont, knew every trick that came with the two feet of snow we'd get in Milwaukee. Building these great snow caves, making snow angels, teaching us to ice-skate, putting these ridiculous-looking skis on the girls and letting them jump over the ridiculous little hump that he built back there. That was a blackberry.

I have remembered for the last few days so many great moments, but one in particular is when we were on vacation up in Vermont where Dad was from. We were at a farm up there. And there were a bunch of cousins and friends, maybe six or seven of us. And Dad would just throw us pop-ups out in this open field next to this barn near the house. You could just do that forever. But the other kids would start to lose interest, so six dwindled down to five, four, three, and then it was just me and one other guy. We said, "Maybe about ten steps this time. Throw one I can dive for." Then it was just me and him.

I said, "Just one more." He knew it wasn't the last one. "Hey, just one more, Dad."

Asking for just one more throw is what I've been feeling for the past few days. Just one more. One more day. One more hour. One more minute.

He had these habits and sayings around the house that became blackberries for us, things we've laughed about through the years. Anytime you were at dinner, it was, "Chew it up small." "Dad, we're having soup, c'mon." "No horseplay," he'd say. No horseplay at the table, no horseplay in the car, no horseplay that's any fun. "Drive slow." That was a big one, especially when we all became drivers. "Drive slow." He got on my mom once back when the speed limit was 55 because she was going 56. "Hey, lead foot."

He passed on his rare abilities in household repair to all of us. Mom likes to say he's the only man in America who's never been in a Home Depot. My dad's answer to everything when it came to household repair was a can of three-in-one oil. And it didn't matter what the problem was. Three-in-one oil did the trick. Squeaky hinges? Three-in-one. Storm damage? Three-in-one. He used it on my baseball glove. It was, "Here's some three-in-one. Throw it in there." Out of salad dressing? Three-in-one oil.

I like to call him a sportscaster with a speech impediment. He couldn't say no. Charity golf tournaments, speaking engagements, you name it, he was there. Mom lost track of all the nights he was away from the house, away from the kids, speaking. "Dad's not here tonight. He's out speaking to a group of dads about spending time with their kids."

Dad read about a kid named Ricky Haygood who got paralyzed a long time ago because of a football injury, and they became lifelong friends. Ricky lived in south Georgia. Nobody brought Dad's attention to it. He just read it and fell in love with it. He had such a heart. And it didn't matter—we would be on vacation or he'd be speaking in south Georgia, and it was always, "Hey, hold on, we're going to stop by and see Ricky." We'd be on our way back from Florida and we'd stop by to see Ricky. The Haygoods made Dad an honorary member of their family. It was that way with Kelly Hayes too in her wheelchair. I remember something Dad used to say on the radio: "I'm going to say hello to all the shut-ins. I know you can't get to the ballpark, but we're thinking about you."

He was a constant source of encouragement, so proud of Chris and Dawn as they pursued the teaching profession. I went the less cerebral route, into television. But you know, when he and my mom were coming back from Florida once and I had just started my career in Macon, anchoring the news, they looked at their watches as they were driving up 75 and said, "Hey, you know what? It's almost six o'clock. If we stop around here somewhere, we can watch the six o'clock news on channel 13 in Macon." This is a true story. They pulled into a hotel down there around Warner Robins or Unadilla or somewhere that got WMAZ. It's two minutes to six. They get out of their car, go inside, and tell the guy behind the desk they need a room for a half hour. I can just picture that clerk saying, "All right, Ernie." He said, "No, I want to watch the news, really."

The greatest thing I've ever done or will ever do in my career is work with my dad. They made that happen on SportSouth in the midnineties. To sit in that booth with a man who is respected by so many, loved by so many fans, it was the greatest thing anybody has ever done for my career. I want to thank Garland Simon—she's here with Ned—and it was her idea to have us work together. For me, it was a chance to sit shoulder to shoulder with that legend and try not to embarrass him.

There are so many folks who don't have that relationship with their dad, and I feel for you. I talk to guys who say, "I haven't talked to my dad in years. He and I just don't see eye to eye." I never took for granted the blessing it was to have that kind of relationship with my dad. He was the best man in my wedding, my best friend. He simply taught me everything I needed to know about how to work, how to be a dad, how to be a husband. If you gave me eighty-seven years and sixty-three years married to the same woman, I'd take it.

There are certain blackberries in my dad's life.

Those Marine Corps reunions. He was so proud. I remember him telling us all, "I won the war. We were losing when I went in. And when I came out, we had won."

High school reunions he and Mom would go to in Brattleboro, Vermont. They'd have these parades, and Mom and

Dad would be the grand marshals. I'm surprised you haven't seen it; it was on cable. Those were huge blackberry moments.

Those vacations on Anna Maria Island, which we took as kids, which Mom and Dad continued to do. I'd see them out there in their beach chairs watching the sunset. Dad's got one hand on a gin and tonic and the other in my mom's hand.

The Wednesday night dinner club. I must have met five hundred people yesterday who were in that Wednesday night dinner club. That was a blackberry.

The workouts at the rehab center. I tried to hammer home to Dad, "Don't tell me you're going to rehab. It sounds very old. Tell me you're going to go work out." So he'd say, "Mom and I are going to go work out." One of his buddies actually said, "Your dad and I used to pump iron."

The chance he had to work at Enable of Georgia. Helping special-needs adults lead productive lives was huge for my dad, a huge blackberry for him.

For all of us the last few days, there was no greater blackberry than Embracing Hospice—the facility where he spent his last days, a place that is staffed 24/7 by absolute angels who know exactly what to say and when to say it. Their care and concern just floor you.

On behalf of our family—Mom Lois, Dawn and Rebecca, Chris and Jackie, Cheryl and Eric, Maggie, Michael and Ashley and Carmen and Allison, thank you for being here. I don't know when we'll see him again, but I know we will.

And while I don't know exactly what heaven is going to be like, I hope there's baseball. And I hope there are blackberries.

3

The Girl at the Bank

STOP ME IF YOU'VE HEARD the one about the Macon, Georgia, bank teller working her way through college who sold her clarinet so she could take her soon-to-be ex-boyfriend out for one last dinner. Oh, you haven't heard that one? True story. I was the soon-to-be ex-boyfriend. The bank teller would somehow turn out to be my wife. Let's step back a few years, and perhaps you'll gain an understanding of how that bizarre chain of events unfolded. I make no promises you will, but here goes.

So I'm a freshman at the University of Georgia in Athens with a love of baseball handed down by my dad, and I'm going to try out for the UGA baseball team. You've heard about guys who spend their junior and senior years of high school going home after school to find letters from colleges and universities drooling over the prospect of having them attend their schools on an athletic scholarship. Now I was a pretty good player at Marist High School in Atlanta, but never did I go to the mailbox and find, amid the bills addressed to my parents or the *Time* and *Newsweek* and *Good House-keeping* magazines, anything resembling one of those letters.

If I was going to keep the dream alive of one day following my dad into the major leagues, I would have to "walk on" at Georgia and be one of the few nonscholarship players on the team. Well, it happened. I made the team and would wear the red and black of the Bulldogs as a reserve first baseman in the 1975 season. It was an incredible experience. Our head coach, Jim Whatley, was a Georgia legend, and he was retiring at season's end, so I was a member of his last team. Just being around those guys every day—listening to their stories, making road trips around the Southeastern Conference, and getting to play the game I loved—was beyond special. I also grew up a lot being in the company of upperclassmen, a couple of whom were already married. I was getting a real-world perspective while still trying to figure out how to find my way around a sprawling campus.

We had a good team and won the Eastern Division of the Southeastern Conference. I played a minuscule role in that success. In fact, if there's a word you have in mind for a contribution that was *less* than minuscule, you just go ahead and use that. The numbers tell the story: 18 at bats, 2 hits, 1 RBI. That wasn't in a week or a month. Those were my totals for the year. Look out, big leagues. Four months later, with a new head coach in place, fall workouts began, and inside a week, for me, they ended. Dream over.

My mom and dad always stressed the idea of having a plan B, and I always told myself that if this baseball thing didn't work out, I would work toward becoming an English teacher and a baseball coach. Dad was never one to push me toward his line of work as a broadcaster, but having spent so many years watching him do a job he so obviously loved, I gave the idea of a media career some serious thought too. A part-time job delivering sports updates on the campus radio station, WUOG, cemented the deal. I changed majors from English to journalism, I got a job at an honest-to-goodness commercial radio station (WAGQ-FM) that paid actual money, and I was hooked. When I graduated in 1978, job one was, well, to find job one in television.

Now we're sort of, gradually, meandering into the Macon, Georgia, bank teller story. I had already failed miserably while auditioning for a TV sports job in Albany, Georgia. Remember the movie *Airplane!* when the actor Robert Hays, playing Ted Striker, takes the controls of that jet? Remember the sweat pouring down his face and drenching his shirt? That was me, times ten, at least.

I had slinked back home to my apartment in Athens with my tail between my legs only to discover that WMAZ, channel 13 in Macon, was offering me a chance to audition for a spot as one of its news anchors. I followed up the Albany disaster with a better effort. And really, anything I did would have been better. Apparently, it was good enough, because all of a sudden viewers were looking at the new anchor of 13 News at 11. He's Ernie Johnson Jr., a recent college graduate who appears to be no more than fifteen years old, who has apparently perfected the art of the monotone delivery and makes lots of mistakes reading the news. But I was so far past cloud nine I'd lost count.

My on-air duties extended beyond the studio in what I can only say was an unexpected way. In the course of my training at the Grady College of Journalism at UGA, my professors had stressed that if you're working in news, you don't stray into, for instance, commercials. It could cause a conflict with your journalistic integrity if a business you're promoting should come under investigation. How do you report on that during the evening news if you're somehow tied to the company? And besides—you're a newsman now; you're not pitching products. So imagine my surprise when in the first month of my employment, the news director, a very nice man who had been at the station for longer than I had been alive, called me in to tell me that I was needed at Barney A. Smith Lincoln Mercury at 1:00 that afternoon.

I assumed there was some kind of feature story in the works but was then told I'd be shooting a commercial at the used-car lot there. I laughed. He didn't. "But how about journalistic integrity? How about news standards? You don't see Dan Rather doing commercials on CBS . . . C'mon!" I could hear my college professors Bill Martin and Marcus Bartlett saying, "Atta boy, Ernie. Go get 'em." But this is what I got back from the station: "Well, we don't quite have the budget here to hire news anchors and commercial talent, so you get to do both."

So if you watched our newscasts in those days, there's a pretty good chance you'd see me reporting on a house fire, a city council meeting, and the latest employment numbers in the first news block. Then we'd go to a commercial break, and after a quick dip to black, yours truly would reappear, earnestly imploring you to "come to the used-car lot at Barney A. Smith Lincoln Mercury. They've got a great supply of late-model used cars for any of your family's needs!" Or you might see me walking the aisles excitedly declaring, "The windows and doors shop at W-Supply has everything you need to make your house look brand-new again!" Or, and this was my personal favorite, standing outside Tommy's Recaps, which specialized in putting new tread on old tires, delivering the catchy phrase "Tommy's Recaps—they save you dollars . . . and that makes sense." Sheesh. But please don't get me wrong here. I loved that job, despite the whole commercial thing. I was learning every aspect of the business. And I was working with great people who took pride in showing kids like me the ropes, and I'm forever in their debt for that. They were people like George Jobin. He was the sports director and became my closest friend. That happens when someone knows that for the first time in your life you're missing Thanksgiving dinner with your family because you have to work. And so you have a seat at their table before heading to the studio.

And there were people outside the confines of the station who were special too. One in particular. Hey, guess what— we've arrived at the Macon, Georgia, bank teller story.

On Friday afternoons, I would drive to the bank just down the street from the studio to deposit my paycheck at the drive-through window. That was where I met the teller Cheryl Deluca. She was beautiful, always seemed to be in a wonderful mood, was even more sarcastic than I was, and always ended our transactions the same way. You know the lollipops that tellers have on hand, presumably to give to kids who have patiently waited in line with Mom or Dad? Well, even though I obviously did not have a child (or perhaps she was insinuating that I was one), Cheryl always put a lollipop in the drawer with my deposit slip. And it had always been crushed into about 314 cherry, lime, or grape pieces. The first time I thought it was just an honest mistake, and then it became a production. She'd ask what flavor I wanted, and then I'd watch her raise her right hand and hear through the teller-to-customer audio system the sound of palm meeting counter, with just a hint of crinkling cellophane thrown in. I would drive away with my pulverized candy, the receipt that indicated my lack of affluence, and this feeling that there was something different about this girl—something carefree, fun, and spontaneous—that attracted me to her.

And there was that question she asked me in the course of one of our early transactions conducted through six inches of bullet-resistant glass as she chuckled at the dollar amount on my paycheck. "So what do you do at WMAZ?" Was she serious? Did she not recognize this big-shot, small-market TV news personality?

"Well . . . I anchor the news."

"Oh, that's nice," she said, adding that she rarely watched TV while working two jobs to put herself through school at Mercer University. This was my kind of girl. Funny, down-to-earth, great work ethic. And since she wasn't glued to the TV, she'd probably never heard me say, "They save you dollars . . . and that makes sense."

It took me a couple months to get up the nerve to ask her out, and when I appeared at her door for our first date, she was stunned to discover I was six foot three, since she had only seen me seated in my luxurious Chevrolet Monza—the one badly in need of a new clutch, an oil change, and a fresh set of tires. But hey, when you're making the kind of coin I was bringing home, there were monthly decisions to make on whether the rent or the power bill would be paid on time. There wasn't money for something as frivolous as auto maintenance.

Cheryl was pursuing a degree in psychology, and when she wasn't studying, or crushing my lollipops at the drive-through window, she was working as an assistant to a local psychologist. In her precious few free moments, she was spending weekends with a teenaged girl as part of the Big Brothers Big Sisters program. Yes, I was impressed. We dated for several months until I had a chance to climb the career ladder and move from Macon (TV market size 135 out of roughly 220 in the country) to Spartanburg, South Carolina (market number 35).

We hit that "Well, I guess this is it" moment. She had to finish school. I had to take the next career step. On the Wednesday before the weekend I was going to pack up and leave for Spartanburg, she called to say we should go out for dinner that Friday. Her treat. Leo's was one of Macon's most popular restaurants, one of those special occasion places, and since I didn't really have any special occasions to celebrate, I had never been there. That and the fact that it was really expensive. Neither one of us could really afford to go there, but on this night, our last date, we were going.

There was a lot of talk between us about the time we'd spent together and where we saw our lives going, and as I dipped another bite of lobster into the silver cup of melted butter in front of me, this happened:

Me: So ... um ... uh ... how the heck are you planning to pay for this?

Her: Well ... um ... uh ... I sold my clarinet.

Me: Your clarinet? You have ... I mean, you *had* a clarinet?

Her: Yeah. I was in the high school band and still had it in my closet until a couple days ago. I wanted to take *you* out this time, so I went to a pawnshop and sold my clarinet.

Me: (*silently to myself*) I think I might be in love.

On that very cool note, I moved to Spartanburg, and it was probably six months before Cheryl and I spoke again. During that time, on my trips home, Mom or Dad would ask about my love life or lack of it, and my response was always the same. "Guys, I think I blew it when I left the girl at the bank. She was the one." So six months after the "lobster and clarinet dinner," I picked up the phone in Spartanburg and called Cheryl in Macon to see if she might want to meet up in Atlanta and go to the Dan Fogelberg concert. I laid it all out for her:

Me: Nice, fun evening . . . some laid-back acoustic tunes with great lyrics . . . no pressure . . . just hang out and see each other again. Could be some fun . . . whatcha think?

Her: Somebody already asked me to the Dan Fogelberg concert.

Me: (*silently to myself*) Well, that went well.

This will sound incredibly corny, but when I hung up, my mind immediately went to a Fogelberg song. "Once upon a Time" describes that feeling of knowing you met the perfect woman but somehow let her go, and now you're sitting in your one-bedroom Spartanburg apartment, staring at your rented furniture, your shag carpet, and your harvest-gold Trimline phone, and just kicking yourself.

Now before you label me a loser or start a petition to have my man card rescinded, let me capsulate the rest of the story. I kept calling. She eventually agreed to let me come and see her in Macon. Hmm, maybe I hadn't blown it with the girl from the bank after all. We started dating again. I was driving four hours from Spartanburg to Macon just about every weekend. I told her I thought we should get married. She agreed. We did, in 1982. The end. Actually, the beginning.

There is no way I could have foreseen, even with the qualities that attracted me to her in the first place, the impact Cheryl would have on the world around her. The way she gave her time on the weekends for one teenaged girl named Tina in the Big Sisters program gave me just a glimpse of her heart to be a positive influence in a life that had more of its share of negatives. It was that heart that years later would lead us down the road of adoption, not once but four times. It was that heart that would take her into a leadership role with Metro Atlanta Recovery Residences (MARR), a nonprofit devoted to helping women break the chains of drug and alcohol addiction.

Cheryl went back to school in her forties to earn her master's degree as a licensed professional counselor. She assumed a leadership position with the women's program at MARR, and her influence was profound. For seven years she was counselor, confidant, disciplinarian, and friend to so many women who had lost everything to addiction—husbands, families, careers—women who had, in short, lost their way.

Coming from me, that description of her influence might sound like a proud husband heaping praise on his wife. But the words that follow come from those she tirelessly shepherded through some of life's deepest valleys. They were written by those who rediscovered their way thanks in large part to my wife's devotion to the cause. They were compiled in a framed thank-you gift that hangs in a hallway in our home amid years of family photos and mementos.

"The visible, palpable way she cares for women is
   phenomenal."

"Everything she shares is important to my recovery."

"Taught me skills I will use my entire life."

"I hang on her every word."

"She knows what I think and feel before I do."

"She is tough yet compassionate."

"Radiates power and love."

"She is all that!"

It was that heart, obvious to anyone who has the good fortune to interact with her, that led Street Grace, another nonprofit organization, to ask Cheryl to lead the campaign to raise awareness about the issue of sex trafficking of children in the Atlanta area. She would eventually become the group's CEO, and she would take the effort well beyond the city limits of Atlanta to states around the Southeast.

Anything of real, true, life-changing significance that our family has been involved with has come mainly from the heart of Cheryl Deluca-Johnson. I'm a sportscaster. She's a world changer. I have been blessed to be along for the ride.

One year for our anniversary (sorry I can't be more specific, but thirty-four years become a blur sometimes) I wanted to get her something different yet special. Something that demonstrated a degree of thought not often associated with roses, a piece of jewelry, or a gift card to Walmart. This would be a challenge, but I found a store that had just what I was looking for. This was not a place that would offer to do the gift wrapping for me while I waited. I handled that in my own rudimentary way, which as always resulted in several spots where tape was easily visible. And I found an anniversary card—not one of those cards emblazoned with beautiful flowers and flowery prose but a simple, no-frills, little-artwork, your-own-message-to-be-written-on-the-inside kind of card. I left the wrapped present and the card on the kitchen counter so they would be the first things she saw when she walked in from work that afternoon, and I watched from the kitchen table as she read what I had written: "Happy anniversary. I think I owe you one of these."

And then with some difficulty, given the roll and a half of tape I had used, she unwrapped her present. A brand-new . . . clarinet. You know those blackberry moments I like to talk about? They're treasures. Her buying me dinner in Macon with the funds from selling her clarinet was certainly one I'll never forget. And this new clarinet was one for her . . . and for somebody I've never met. A couple hours later Cheryl came to me with a request. "Would it be okay if I donated the clarinet to the high school band program? I'm sure there's a kid out there who can't afford one, and this would be such a cool surprise."

My kind of girl.

4

We Have Company

IT IS THE SINGLE MOST-ASKED QUESTION by college students who have chosen to major in journalism/broadcasting: "What advice would you give an aspiring journalist/broadcaster?" When I was in school, I had a three-step approach when meeting somebody who was working in TV. Shake their hand, look 'em in the eye, and fire off the question. I was an annoying student. Then I'd walk away and scribble down those nuggets of career advice.

For a guy who asked that question a lot, these days I love *getting* that question. It's a chance to pass on my dad's advice about being yourself and working harder than the next guy, and I get to share what I've experienced in terms of the value of good writing, solid reporting, and learning to do a variety of jobs.

That was the great thing about Macon and Spartanburg. I did everything—shoot, edit, and produce stories. I would sit with producers and learn how they formatted a newscast. So when I'm asked that question, a part of my answer is always, "Be versatile." I liken it to spring training in baseball. When a manager has to trim his roster to twenty-five players as the season is about to start, and he's down to that last spot, who gets it? Often it's the guy who can do more than one thing. He can play both corners of the infield, maybe some outfield, and even fill in if the starting catcher gets hurt. And he's a switch-hitter. By the same token, when a news director needs to make a hire and sees somebody who can report in the field, shoot video, edit, and even anchor a newscast, that guy is going to have an edge over somebody who's one-dimensional. Oh, and there's another thing I tell the "aspiring" crowd: never underestimate the value of timing and luck.

In the summer of 1983, I'd been a general assignment news reporter at WSB-TV in Atlanta for just over a year. A new news director had just been appointed. Rabun Matthews came down from Washington, DC, and on his first day, I was filling in for one of our vacationing sports reporters. The next day Rabun summoned me to his office. As I weaved my way through the cubicles of my fellow reporters in the newsroom, past the assignment desk, I had no idea what awaited me. Did he just want to introduce himself? Was this something all the reporters were doing? Should I start boxing up all my belongings? None of the above. He asked me if I'd be interested in moving from news to sports, and if so, I could be the new weekend sports anchor. Just like that (I'm snapping my fingers for effect) my career path was forever changed.

Timing and luck. At least that's the way I viewed it at that very moment. It would be fourteen years before my view of timing and luck was transformed into a wondrous view of how God orchestrates every move in my life. How God connects the dots in ways I cannot fathom. Hold on to that thought. In TV parlance, it's what we call a tease. More to come on that story a little later. Stay tuned.

It is going to sound very stupid when I say this (kind of my comfort zone), but the toughest thing about being the weekend sports anchor is you have to work weekends. That means, of course, that when all of your friends are planning fun stuff for Saturday and Sunday, your wife is telling them, "Oh, that sounds great, but Ernie's working, so we'll have to pass."

I did, however, get a Saturday off in September 1984, though it was unplanned. It was the twenty-ninth, and I was just about to get out of bed and get ready to go downtown for the Georgia Tech–Clemson football game when Cheryl, then eight months pregnant with our first child, informed me this pregnancy would not be nine months in duration. We were the proud parents of Eric Deluca Johnson at 4:00 that afternoon. And honestly, we were clueless.

That's the thing about being a parent for the first time. You can try to prepare for it and read baby books and talk to your friends who have been there, but you're basically just learning on the fly. And it is glorious. Until it isn't. Sometimes you're downright scared. You can't figure out why this two-month-old can't hold down any food, and you're spending your first Thanksgiving as a family in the hospital. And a doctor is operating on him for something called pyloric stenosis, which you learn affects a lot of firstborn males. The opening between the stomach and the small intestine thickens, and food has nowhere to go but on your favorite shirt again and again and again. Eventually, you start wearing your least favorite shirt because you know how it's gonna wind up. But the doctors fixed our little guy, and we went merrily along, taking a thousand pictures of Eric doing everything and doing nothing for two and a half years until his little sister came along.

Eric was a lot like me growing up. In the old home movies my dad took of us in the fifties and sixties, with no sound and lots of camera shaking, I was rarely without a bat and ball. I absolutely loved baseball, and Eric was drawn by that same magnet. When I watched him play, I couldn't help but think about my own childhood and my dream of playing in the majors like my dad had. Eric loved the game too and was good at it. And that's where things can get a little sideways if you're not careful. I've seen too many dads put too many unrealistic expectations on their sons, and suddenly, they're not playing because *they* love the game but because *you* do. Before you know it, you've turned into the Little League manager's nightmare: the Little League parent.

"My son should be playing shortstop."

"My son should be hitting leadoff."

"My son should be pitching."

"You're not using my boy the right way. He's got big league talent, and he'll never get there if you're calling the shots."

My dad was never like that. Thank God. He was a great teacher of the game, having played it at the highest level, and he was always helping me improve, but he let the coaches coach and respected the difficulty of their jobs. I tried to be the same way with Eric, but man, it's tough, isn't it, dads? You want so badly for your child to succeed, but you can unwittingly put so much pressure on him that the baseball field is transformed from a wonderland into a torture chamber, and a throwing error or a rally-killing strikeout means a lecture on the way home. It's dangerous territory.

I always admired my father's patience and restraint when watching me try to follow in his big league footsteps, and I was grateful, too, that he never made it a requirement that I play baseball. If I had wanted to hang it up, I could have, but that wasn't going to happen. It was in my blood, and I played the game until reality set in during my second year at the University of Georgia. I was grateful for having played my freshman year, but being cut as a sophomore, while it disappointed me, did not shock me. I simply didn't have the talent to make it a career.

Eric was a better player at his age than I was. I'll admit that, and there was a part of me—the hopeful father part—that could see him making it farther than I had. I was disappointed when after making his high school team as a tenth grader he told me he'd had enough. The game just wasn't fun anymore. He didn't want to report to school an hour before classes started to work out with the pitchers. The game had lost its magic for him. He had hinted during tryouts that he was tired of playing, but Cheryl and I had urged him to stick it out—not to quit—thinking that if he was good enough to make the squad, his outlook would change. It didn't, and that's when we had our talk, and he had his say, and grudgingly I said okay.

Was it the right decision on my part as a dad? Should I have forced him to keep playing? My dad wouldn't have done that to me, and I wasn't going to do that to Eric. You know what made it tough? Our bloodlines. Growing up as

Ernie Johnson Jr. brought its own set of pressures. I heard the talk as a kid. "The only reason Ernie made the all-star team is because his dad is the Braves' broadcaster." Eric was going through some of that same stuff, with a grandfather who was adored by baseball fans and a father who was a sportscaster. He had every right in the world to wonder if he was just supposed to play because of those ties. I didn't want him burdened with that. I told him, "Big Guy never pushed me to play ball, and he didn't push me to pursue a career in broadcasting, Eric. I did those things because I was passionate about both. Now here's what you do. Find what you're passionate about—what makes your heart beat a little faster—and then go after it with all you've got." I don't know what other dads would have done, but that's what this dad did, with no regrets. And you know what? These days I can still find a blackberry when we pull out our gloves and the two of us—the sixty-year-old dad and the thirty-two-year-old son—step out on the lawn and play catch.

While I witnessed Eric's birth at Cheryl's bedside, that wouldn't be the case with Maggie in April 1987. She would be delivered by C-section, and so I was told I'd have to leave the room at some point. I guess the last thing a doctor and his team need to be doing while they're delivering a baby is scraping Dad off the floor. "All right, Mr. Johnson, it's time for you . . ." I'm assuming the rest of that sentence was "to leave the room, and we'll come and get you a little later" because I was already in the hallway. In time, I was invited back in to gaze at my baby daughter for the first time. I had certainly heard all the stories about how little girls get their fathers wrapped around their little fingers, and from my experience, I can verify that it is indeed true. It takes forty-three seconds. So in the span of four years, seven months, and nineteen days from our wedding day, the Johnson family was complete. Cheryl and I had decided having a boy and a girl was pretty much all we could ask for, not to mention handle.

That all changed a few years later.

I came home from work late one afternoon in the fall of 1990, and Cheryl posed this question: "You know what we need to do?" I assumed this was some type of dinner-related question to which I would respond that chicken or fish would be nice. It was not a dinner-related question. "I think we need to adopt a child from Romania. I watched the 20/20 story on ABC the other night and just cried at what's happening to kids over there. How would you feel about going there to adopt one?" I was not prepared for this line of questioning. Nor was I prepared for the heartbreaking stories I would then read. Romanian dictator Nicolae Ceaușescu had mandated that the country reverse its low birthrate and to that end had outlawed contraception, even promising "benefits" to women who gave birth to at least five children.

Much of Romania was impoverished, and many children were abandoned and sent to orphanages that soon became overcrowded and under-maintained. If a child had a handicap, he or she would wind up in one of the so-called Homes for the Deficient and Unsalvageable. When the Ceaușescu regime was overthrown in 1989 and the dictator and his wife were executed, the world would learn of Romania's forgotten and neglected children and of the horrendous conditions in which they were living. And dying. We decided to try in some small way to help.

If you've ever been through the process of adoption, you know there is a mountain of paperwork. We filled out every form. There are home studies by adoption agencies to determine if you're qualified to adopt. We went through a series of those interviews. In the spring of 1991, we were given the green light, found a group of other would-be adoptive parents who were planning a May trip to Romania, and signed up. Our intent was to adopt a baby girl in the eight-month-old range with no permanent handicaps. Our hope was that doctors here in the States could fix whatever illness she might be suffering from and give her a fresh start.

Cheryl would go to Romania with the group we had met. I would stay home and take care of Eric, now six, and Maggie, now four. I would have reinforcements in the child care department with my mom and dad and Cheryl's parents, Lou and Joan Deluca, who by the way are just about the greatest in-laws in the history of in-laws. On nights when I had to work, one of those sets of grandparents would take care of the kids.

Cheryl packed for what we believed would be a month-long trip, tops. It turned out to be closer to two months. The adoption process was an exercise in international red tape and ever-changing rules. To try to circumvent some of that, my wife, on the advice of the trip organizers, brought a suitcase filled with bribes—cartons of cigarettes, bottles of whiskey, and more cosmetics than you'll find at a Miss Universe pageant. They would all be used before her journey was over.

Cheryl left for Romania on May 16 and settled into a small apartment in Bucharest. After enlisting the help of a cab driver named Sorin Decu, who also served as her interpreter, she made her first visit to an orphanage in a village outside Bucharest. On May 21, on one of those rare occasions when we were able to secure a phone line, Cheryl detailed that visit for me. As she waited in the lobby, a nurse brought out a child. It was not an eight-month-old girl but a boy, not quite three years old. He had been abandoned in a park at birth. He could not walk. He could not speak. On the other end of the phone, my wife was having trouble speaking. She was in tears.

"Hon, I met this little boy today. The first child I saw. The nurse told me, 'Do not take. Boy is no good.' Ern, he has so many issues, he's so much more than we said we could handle, but I don't know if I can go the rest of my life wondering what happened to him."

Her words hung there, demanding a response, for ten seconds, with neither of us speaking. Sometimes you are captured, even on a scratchy telephone line halfway around the world, not by the words you're hearing but by *how* they are spoken. Those words were coming from some inner recess of Cheryl's heart, some place not easily accessed, some place for which only an abandoned, hopeless Romanian orphan had the key. Suddenly, all the things we had talked about and all the things we had written in the required adoption paperwork about the severity of a child's condition we were willing to take on became secondary.

"Then bring him home."

His name was Aurel Mihai Urzicaneau. Mihai is the Romanian version of Michael, and that's what we would call him. Getting him home would require patience, determination, and resolve. Three qualities my wife has in abundance. We hit numerous roadblocks in the process. In fact, at one point, Romania put a temporary stop to all adoptions, but since Cheryl had already started the process, our case was allowed to continue. And those bribes—they came in handy. Can't get your hands on the necessary paperwork to complete the next step in the process? Give the clerk a bottle of whiskey or a carton of Kools, and suddenly a form that was supposed to take four days is there the next afternoon. Want the nurse to give Michael a little more to eat? One of those American makeup kits did the trick. Cheryl learned quickly that if you're going to play the adoption game in Romania, sadly, you have to play by certain rules. She's my hero.

Meanwhile, back in Atlanta, I was preparing a homecoming gift for Cheryl. I had decided to chronicle the events at home as Eric and Maggie and I did life without Mom for nearly two months. I would scribble down notes every day about what we did, and then late at night when the kids were in bed, I would compose "How I Spent My Summer Vacation." It told a tale of blackberry moments as well as nights of utter frustration and even an episode that perfectly illustrated the fact that Dad had passed down his handyman gene to me . . . unfortunately. Here are some excerpts.

May 21, 1991

I left the Techwood studios a little after two in the morning and just drove, windows down, stereo not quite blasting. I drove to my old neighborhood and saw the house I lived in when our family moved to Atlanta. Drove down Roswell Road past the apartment complex where a drunk driver clobbered me and my sister Chris one night almost twenty years ago. Drove past Cheryl's old neighborhood in Norcross and all the while just tried to put all of this into perspective. While I want to believe that things will go smoothly for Cheryl over there, I don't want to take anything for granted. While I already consider Aurel Mihai a member of our family, I'll truly believe it when I see him and Cheryl at the airport.

May 29, 1991

Major faux pas by yours truly today. Eric went back to school after yesterday's sickness, but I failed to check the calendar and thus failed to attend kindergarten awards day. Eric didn't mention it until after taking his bath tonight, and then he proceeded to take from his backpack the certificates he had won while the other parents watched. Eric won the reading award and the citizenship award for his class, and I wasn't there. All I could do was conjure up these images of Eric walking to the podium to pick up his awards when his name was called and scanning the audience for me and Mags. He was so grown up not to make a big deal out of it. And to cap it off, after I read a couple books to the kids before bed, Eric came downstairs with the Best Reader Award for me.

July 1, 1991

It was now time to start getting things ready in earnest, and the first task was to assemble the crib used by Eric and Maggie for Michael. Feeling the need for a work area that would be spacious, I chose the den despite the fact that the crib would go in Eric's room upstairs. I figured, not having taken the time to measure, that the crib would fit through the door of Eric's room. I started at 12:45, and within fifteen minutes, I had finished . . . I thought. Actually, the sides of the crib were on backward, so I disassembled it and within twenty-five minutes had reassembled it.

My success was diminished somewhat when Maggie asked me why I hadn't just put it together in Eric's room (just what I needed to hear from a four-year-old). Eric helped me carry the crib upstairs. I would have had an easier time fitting a 1976 El Camino through that bedroom door. So at 1:55, I was outside Eric's room again disassembling the crib. After moving all the parts into Eric's room, I put the crib back together, but now the frame that holds the mattress would not fit. So I made the decision to once again take it all apart. It was 3:00, and I was back to square one. Shortly before 4:00, I finally finished. I stood back and admired my work, disregarding the fact that just about anybody else in the country not only would have completed the job but also would have watched *Gone with the Wind* and been pretty deep into *Crime and Punishment* in the same period of time.

July 5, 1991

Cheryl's not back yet, but she will be tomorrow, so this will be the final chapter. The kids and I hit Toys "R" Us today for crib sheets, a car seat, and a couple toys for themselves, and I couldn't stop thinking about the next day—what it will be like when Cheryl and Michael get off the plane. We plan to have vanilla wafers for Michael and flowers for Cheryl, and there will be family members there, and it's just gonna be . . . nice.

Cheryl is on her way home now and called today from Frankfurt. I could tell by the first words out of her mouth that she was in the best mood she'd been in since May 16.

There was a sense of total relief and accomplishment that I couldn't have been imagining. She had done it, and in twenty-four hours, she could begin telling me detail by detail just what it was like over there. That's really the story worth telling. Welcome home.

On Saturday, July 6, Cheryl's plane touched down in Atlanta, and now all the Johnsons and all the Delucas would get their first up close look at this kid named Michael, whom we had only seen in photographs. The doors at the international concourse were those automatic kind that slide open and shut, and we really couldn't see through them. So every time they slid open, we'd sit up or stand up and hope that Cheryl would appear. There were a lot of false starts.

Then the doors slid open and out walked this incredibly courageous woman pushing a stroller that appeared to be about as frail as the passenger it carried. Everybody was hugging and kissing and crying and . . . gazing at this blond-haired boy. A month shy of his third birthday, Michael was tiny and silent, aside from making a few indiscernible sounds. These skinny legs were sticking out from a pair of shorts, and the white socks on his feet had slid down near his heels. He wasn't wearing shoes because he couldn't wear shoes. His left foot was turned in at the ankle at nearly a ninety-degree angle. He was passed from one family member to another like a gift that everybody wants to see on Christmas morning.

And what a gift he was.

And now a footnote to this Romanian adventure. I mentioned that Cheryl was aided in her journey by a cab driver named Sorin Decu. He took her wherever she needed to go.

He was able to break through the language barrier at every step and give Cheryl the answers to the myriad questions she had.

After Cheryl was back home, we heard from Sorin that he was attempting to immigrate to the United States. He had the proper work papers and was ready to travel to the United States while his wife and two children stayed behind. Once Sorin was able to establish himself in the American workforce and in time become a citizen, he would be able to bring his family over. It would be a two-year process. For the first six months of his US stay, I guess you can say we adopted him too.

We turned one of the rooms in the basement into his home. He stayed with us, working every day, eating at our kitchen table, even babysitting Michael so Cheryl and I could go out for dinner every now and then. In time, Sorin saved enough money to afford a place of his own, and it felt as if one of our own kids was moving out.

Sorin stayed in touch, letting us know how the process of bringing his family to the United States was going and inviting us to the Romanian church he had discovered. And when we attended his citizenship ceremony, it was as if we were celebrating one of our kids' graduations. Eventually, his perseverance was rewarded, and he welcomed his wife and kids to the United States as they left their homeland for a whole new life. Two years later Sorin and his wife welcomed another son into the world.

They named him Michael.

5

Love You Too

THAT DATE, JULY 6, when Michael arrived in the United States, became a day our family would celebrate every year, but not just because of our new Romanian import. You'll remember our original intent was to adopt a baby girl, and the prospect of having a little sister around the house was something four-year-old Maggie was off-the-charts excited about. And while she and Eric were absolutely wonderful with Michael upon his arrival, Cheryl and I heard incessantly over the next couple years from our only daughter that she would like to lose that "only" label. It was an idea Cheryl and I had brought up in passing, but it was back burner stuff. We had too much going on with Michael's health to even consider expanding our family.

Much of Michael's first year was spent at various doctors' offices and hospitals. The casting and recasting of his lower left leg over the course of a few months eventually removed the limb's sharp right turn at the ankle, and it looked, well, normal. But his digestive system was far from that. He had been given little, if any, solid food in the orphanage. In fact, we had to basically teach him how to chew. He would take food like those vanilla wafers I'd brought to the airport and just let them dissolve in his mouth before he swallowed. We couldn't tell him how to chew—he couldn't speak and had no understanding of our language. We just had to show him, making exaggerated chewing motions, and in time he caught on.

His system was ravaged by parasites, which required weeks of testing by a gastroenterologist to determine exactly what the problem was and how it could be treated. That process was no treat—I'll leave it at that. And then there were the neurological tests. How severe were the developmental delays? we worried. Would there come a time when we would not be awakened in the morning to the sound of this child rocking on all fours, rhythmically banging his head against the crib? Would he ever speak? These were just a few of the questions we peppered the specialists with for months. The answers were not encouraging. One doctor told us Michael would never talk, would never bond with another person. In short, what we were seeing now was not going to change appreciably.

What did encourage us was that physically Michael was making some progress. He was walking. He didn't put one foot in front of the other but had more of a side-to-side, waddling gait, but hey, considering he had not walked in the first three years of his life, we were thrilled. In fact, the way he moved was kind of similar to the way the legendary manager of the Atlanta Braves, Bobby Cox, would stroll to the mound to make a pitching change. The first time Michael went trick-or-treating with his big brother and sister, we put him in a Braves uniform and wrote the last name Cox and the number 6 on the back of his jersey. It was a hoot. Until it wasn't.

When our pediatrician watched him walk in the hallway of his office, he recommended a visit to a neuromuscular specialist. His suspicions led to surgery—a muscle biopsy that left Michael with a three-inch scar on his left thigh. The diagnosis left us speechless. Michael had Duchenne muscular dystrophy, a genetic disorder in which the muscles gradually weaken and deteriorate. There is no known cure. All we knew about MD was what we'd seen every Labor Day when Jerry Lewis would hold a telethon to raise money for research to help Jerry's kids. Now Michael was one of them.

Because there is no cure, for many of those afflicted, kids are all they will ever be, especially if they have Duchenne. Cheryl and I were numb, confused, heartbroken, you name it. Yet we were determined to do what we had set out to do in the first place—make this child's life a better one than what he had before. Friends would sometimes say something that I found curious, but then with repetition it really bothered me. The statement was usually prefaced with "I'm so sorry to hear about Michael." Then the speaker would continue, "I guess if you guys had known he had muscular dystrophy, you wouldn't have adopted him." Nothing could have been further from the truth. In as understanding a tone as I could muster, I would explain that we had adopted Michael not with an eye on what he would *become* but for who he *was*, a neglected, forgotten child who deserved another chance.

We knew he had a variety of problems, but we knew nothing of his birth parents, who had abandoned him shortly after his birth, or if doctors had ever taken the time to truly diagnose everything that was going on. All we knew was that he needed a home, and we were going to provide it, no matter what the doctors in the States would eventually discover about his issues. And to take it to another level, in my view, we had no guarantees that something catastrophic wouldn't happen to Eric or Maggie. Would we then take the stance that we should never have had them in the first place? Never. We would face that crisis head-on and do whatever we had to do to get through it. And that's what we were going to do with Michael.

Now back to Maggie and her never-ending quest for a little sister. After about a year and a half, we had settled into a new normal, for lack of a better term, and Cheryl and I were pulled toward the idea of adopting again. There were two ground rules. It was going to be a girl, obviously. And because of Michael's situation and all it entailed, we were not in a position to adopt another child with special-needs. We contacted an agency and went through the same exhausting but necessary regimen of paperwork and home studies used to determine if we were candidates to adopt. We passed the audition and waited for a phone call.

On July 6, 1993, God winked. That's right—July 6— exactly two years to the day that Cheryl had pushed Michael through the international concourse at the Atlanta airport, the adoption agency called Cheryl wondering if we were interested in adopting a baby girl from Paraguay. Timing and luck, right? Cheryl told them she had a phone call to make. I answered the call in St. Louis, where I would be calling the Braves-Cardinals game with my dad the following night. Cheryl jumped right in.

"I just got off the phone with the adoption agency."

"And . . ."

"There's a baby in South America . . . Paraguay. Her name is Carmen Esquivel. She's a healthy six-month-old. They want to know if we're interested. Can you believe we got this call on this day?"

I was shaking with excitement and shaking my head in disbelief. "July 6. Let's go to Paraguay."

Compared with the Romanian adventure Cheryl had endured two years earlier, this was cake. With our two sets of parents again playing the role of babysitters/lifesavers, Cheryl and I went together for a week to the capital city of Asunción. We had already been told that the adoption would not be finalized for three weeks, so our plan was to spend a week there with Carmen and then leave her in the care of a foster mother while we went back to Eric, Maggie, and Michael and waited for word on when to go back.

Arriving on Saturday, we were told by the Paraguayan attorney who was handling the adoption that on Sunday afternoon she would bring Carmen to our hotel. And so on Sunday we waited, and we paced, and we read, and we watched some TV, and we strolled through the hotel's garden area, where among other things we could stare at a caged monkey. Having exhausted our list of things to do to kill time, we paced some more, and Sunday afternoon became Sunday night, and it started pouring. And then, as we stood near the driveway of the Grand Hotel del Paraguay, we saw headlights, and a black sedan with its windshield wipers going full throttle eased to a stop underneath the covered entrance to the hotel.

The attorney emerged from the front seat, opened the door to the backseat, and reached into the child seat. As she stepped toward us, we saw Carmen. And now the tears were pouring. If there's one thing adoption has taught us, it's that we have absolutely no understanding of the capacity to love that resides in the human heart. Just when you think you can't possibly love anybody more than you love your spouse, you have a child, and you tap that reservoir of love. We've learned that reservoir is bottomless. Can somebody please explain to me the instant bond that is formed when you hold a baby for the first time? Didn't think so. But for us, it was unmistakable and unbreakable. We were taking turns holding our new daughter. And amid all the thoughts that were colliding in my head, I thought, "Man, is Maggie gonna be thrilled."

The next four days were filled with doing baby stuff—making her laugh, letting her fall asleep in our arms, pushing her stroller on walks near the hotel or in a shopping area in Asunción, showing her the monkey in the cage, and discovering her insatiable appetite for mashed potatoes. Or as the hotel restaurant waiter Santiago told us in Spanish, "*puree de papas.*" By the end of the week, whenever Santiago saw us coming, he would immediately bring a bowl to the table.

We were dreading Friday, because that's when we would have to give Carmen back until the rest of the adoption paperwork could be finalized in three weeks. I don't need to paint that picture for you—it was a tough morning, saying good-bye to Carmen while the foster mother waited to take her away, but there was no getting around it. The other kids needed us too. So we flew home, eager to share all the pictures we'd taken and the stories we'd collected. And we waited for the phone to ring. When we got the call that everything was official, Cheryl flew solo back to South America while

I stayed with the kids. This time when the attorney handed Carmen to Cheryl, it was for good. Forever.

So now we had this mini United Nations right there in the Atlanta suburb of Suwanee. Let me take just a second to heap some praise on Eric and Maggie. Never did they differentiate between their being our biological kids and Michael and Carmen being adopted. To them, we were simply a family, and their sensitivity to Michael's situation in particular was good for the soul.

They were protective of their little brother and bristled when he would draw stares from other kids who were wondering, without verbalizing it, what was wrong with him. Why was he making noises, walking funny, and sometimes just gazing skyward? Why was he in a stroller when he wasn't a baby? Sometimes we'd catch a glimpse of somebody staring out of the corner of an eye, and we'd just invite them over and tell the *Reader's Digest* version of Michael's story. Maybe, we thought, they'd walk away with at least a bit of an understanding that we're all different in some ways, that there's nothing in writing that says we all have to play by the same rules, that there is value in everyone, not just the physically gifted, or the most popular, or the best looking. If strangers didn't get it, our kids certainly did. And through the years, we marveled at the impact Michael had. His physical limitations were no match for his indomitable spirit.

When Eric and Maggie moved into their teenage years, they volunteered as counselors at a wonderful summer camp an hour outside Atlanta. Camp Twin Lakes in the town of Rutledge welcomed kids with all sorts of illnesses for a week of swimming, horseback riding, canoeing, arts and crafts—all the summer camp staples. One week the camp was reserved for cancer patients, another week for kids with autism, another for young people with diabetes. Then there was our week—"Camp Walk and Roll" for children and teenagers with muscular dystrophy. Eric and Maggie didn't volunteer to take care of Michael there; he already had an annual guardian angel at Twin Lakes, a man by the name of Chuck Otto, who used a week of vacation time every year to go to camp. He became Michael's counselor and his buddy. In the meantime, Eric and Maggie took care of other campers who were dealing with the same things they saw Michael deal with in our home. They pushed wheelchairs, held the hands of those who could still walk, carried kids into and out of the swimming pool, took them to the bathroom, helped them shower. They had become the kind of young people Cheryl and I wanted to brag about, like I just did. And Carmen, though younger than Michael, would demonstrate that same selfless heartbeat as she grew older and Michael began showing more and more the effects of muscular dystrophy. Truly, with each passing day, all of us were living lives increasingly enriched by the boy a Romanian nurse had once said was "no good."

Remember the words of the neurologist who told us Michael would never talk and never bond with people? He was wrong. After years of speech therapy, Michael did speak for the first time, at the age of eight, and then we couldn't shut him up!

One development was especially curious. I cannot for the life of me give you a reason for what started happening, other than to point to one doctor's assessment that Michael had a kind of autistic quality when it came to his memory and his fixation with cars. He would flip through brochures from auto dealerships, and though he could not read, he would look at the pictures and we would tell him what they were: Honda Accord, Ford F-150 pickup, Toyota Sienna minivan—the list goes on and on. If a vehicle was on an American road, Michael knew it from sight. And it was always the first question he would try to piece together when meeting our friends. "What car . . . what you . . . what drive?" And when you answered, you entered his memory bank. The next time you saw him, even a year later, he would rattle off a detailed description. "Jeep Cherokee, black outside, gray cloth inside, has lift back, V-6, 2001." And then there would be a jaw-dropping, stunned silence from the owner of that Jeep.

When he wasn't amazing folks with his memory, he was melting their hearts with three words he'd heard a lot around our house and was particularly fond of saying. "Love you too." You didn't necessarily have to tell him you loved him first; he would say it anyway. This from the kid who was never supposed to bond with others and now had a legion of friends and acquaintances who never missed a chance to spend a few minutes with him.

His spirit, his innocence, and his appreciation of even the smallest kind gesture drew people to him in a way we never could have imagined. Phil Bollier was one of those people who felt that attraction, that pull. His chance meeting with Michael became one of those blackberry moments that would change the course of a basketball team, a high school, and dare I say the world.

Phil was an Indiana high school basketball coach who moved his family south so he could become the varsity coach at the newly opened Mill Creek High School in Hoschton, Georgia, a few miles from our home in Braselton. By this time, Michael had been in a wheelchair for a few years, with muscular dystrophy having stolen his ability to stand. As the school year began in 2004, Michael was driving his motorized chair into a special-needs classroom. The gentle whir of the motor caught Phil's attention as he walked down the hallway, and so he poked his head into the classroom and the two struck up a conversation that centered on, you guessed it, what kind of car the coach drove. Michael got the specs, Phil turned to leave, and Michael hit him with the sledgehammer. "Love you too, Bollier."

That afternoon, after the school bus dropped Michael off and as he drove his chair up the driveway, I checked his backpack and found a note from this coach, Phil Bollier. He loved meeting Michael, it read. And he wanted Michael on his team. Why? Because he wanted his players to learn two things from this kid in a wheelchair. One was maximum effort. He knew how limited Michael was physically but also noticed that he used every ounce of energy he had just to get around. And he wanted them to learn what it meant to have a heart for others. Phil had been pierced by those three words: *Love you too.*

When I shared that note with Cheryl, her mind went immediately to a day years before when we were watching one of Eric's Little League games. Michael, wearing the leg braces he always wore before the wheelchair became a necessity, made his way into the dugout and reached for a bat. As Cheryl was about to scoop him up and bring him back to our lawn chairs behind home plate, he said, "Michael play ball." We knew that being on a team like his big brother was on was never going to be an option. But you know the crazy thing about that moment? While Cheryl and I had already come to grips with it, obviously Michael had not. Apparently, in his view, he was at the ballpark, and his brother was playing. Why not grab a bat? Maybe he had never given up hope, even into his high school years. Maybe he knew something we didn't. And now this—an invitation to be a part of the high school basketball team. We were all in.

In no time at all, Michael had memorized every car driven by every player on the team, and for those who didn't drive yet, well, he knew what their parents drove. For fun in the locker room, they would quiz him, and they'd laugh, and Michael would hit 'em with a "Love you too," and they'd say it in return. And since I was usually in there in case Michael needed something, I got to witness this interaction. It was such a blessing. There were times when Coach Bollier's pregame speech would center on Michael. "How high can you raise your right hand, Michael?" the coach would ask. Michael would try to raise his forearm maybe an inch or two off the armrest for just a moment. "You see, boys, everything he does requires maximum effort on his part. Let's make sure we do the same thing tonight. We hold nothing back. Hey, Michael, thanks for that. Love you too."

"Love you too, Bollier."

"Hey, Chase," the coach would say as he looked at his starting point guard. "Love you too."

"Love you too, Coach."

"Hey, Travis, love you too."

"Love you too, Coach."

Hey, Kyle . . . Jermaine . . . Zach . . . the roll call went on with the same encouragement and the same refrain. And as tip-off approached, twelve players would gather around the kid in the wheelchair. One would gently hold Michael's hands

75

in his, and the others would place theirs on top. "One, two, three . . . Hawks!" And then Mill Creek would take the floor. I'd love to say this team wrote a Hollywood script and roared to the state championship. Truth is, this brand-new school lost more than it won. But some seeds were being planted; some blackberries were being enjoyed and shared, both on that basketball court and in the classroom.

When Phil wasn't coaching, he was teaching, and in all of his classes, he would talk about this kid Michael Johnson and his fondness for those three words. He would talk about sign language and how for a lot of students there is just one sign and it involves the middle finger. Phil would say he had another one that should replace that. To say "I love you" in sign language, the index finger and the pinkie are held straight up, and the thumb is extended horizontally. The index finger is the *I*, and with the thumb it forms an *l* for love. The *u* is formed with the index finger and the pinkie. Phil taught this in his classroom. And for a little added touch, he would tip the index finger right at you to say, "Love you too." You didn't have to wear the cardinal and navy blue of the Mill Creek Hawks to learn from Phil Bollier.

This went on for three seasons, Phil coaching and Michael sitting right behind him in his wheelchair. Now let's be clear—Michael didn't really care about basketball, but he loved being a part of that team, being one of the guys. He would come rolling out of the locker room at halftime and fill me in on what had gone on in there. "What did Coach have to say, Michael?"

"Bollier mad. Break a clipboard." In one game that had gotten pretty physical, the Hawks' center, Spencer, fouled out in the closing minutes. He stormed to the bench, threw a towel, took a seat beside Phil, and buried his head in his hands. Michael attempted to cut the tension. "Spencer drive a Isuzu Rodeo?" There was a pause, and then the big man turned and mustered a half smile and a nod.

"Yeah, Mike . . . Isuzu Rodeo. Love you too."

On the night of the final home game of Michael's senior year, the players who would be graduating were honored in a pregame ceremony. They were introduced individually and walked with their parents to center court. They were cheered and given a gray blanket with their name and number embroidered in cardinal red next to the Mill Creek logo. The last name called was Michael Johnson. Cheryl and I walked behind him as he drove his chair to the middle of the floor. As with the other seniors, there was applause, especially from the student section, and when we looked in that direction, we saw them standing, arms raised toward the rafters, hands forming a now familiar message: the "Love you too" sign they had learned from Phil Bollier—a special basketball coach and an even better man.

Phil makes regular trips overseas, coaching with the group Athletes in Action. They've been to China twice, the Philippines, and Macedonia, just to name a few destinations, and no matter where they go, I always get an email. It's always a team picture of Phil's guys and their opponents standing together. And they all have a hand raised, with the index finger and pinkie pointing to the sky and the thumb horizontal, and I know that Phil's been teaching again. And that is always a blackberry to savor.

6

Inside the NBA

UNSCRIPTED. It's the one word that best describes a television show I've hosted for more than a quarter of a century. I can't even begin to total the number of times I've used that word, sometimes adding "spontaneous" or "freewheeling" when a reporter has asked me to describe *Inside the NBA*. It wasn't always that way. For many years, especially early on when I was doing the show solo, no one in the media was really asking questions about the show. It was not unlike others you'd see covering various sports. It was in large part scripted, designed to deliver the night's highlights in a no-nonsense, straightforward way. Not that there's anything wrong with that—I mean, that was what everybody was doing back in the late 1980s and into the 1990s. As the show evolved and TNT added in-studio analysts such as former NBA player Reggie Theus, former NBA coach Dick Versace, and women's hoops legend Cheryl Miller, we started to stray a bit from the established formula. Still, the show didn't look much different from what other networks were doing.

Things started truly changing in the late 1990s when Turner Sports hired Kenny Smith, a two-time NBA champion with the Houston Rockets whose three-point shooting helped propel the Rockets to their back-to-back titles in 1994 and 1995. Kenny is a New York product with a gift for talking basketball that simply resonates with NBA fans. He speaks their language. When Kenny did a few guest appearances before his retirement, the show's producer, Tim Kiely, and I looked at each other one night and agreed that when his playing days were done, Kenny would be a natural fit for the show. He was. No matter what topic I as the host would throw his way, the Jet, as he was known, would take it and run with it.

We developed a really comfortable chemistry after a couple seasons. The show wasn't just informative; it was downright fun, and people were beginning to take notice. One of those people was Charles Barkley, who after announcing his retirement following the 1999–2000 season, immediately became television's most sought-after free agent.

NBC was the early front-runner for the services of Sir Charles, who had long been the league's best sound bite. As a member of the original Olympic Dream Team in 1992, Charles Barkley had quickly become the team's top personality on a team that had its share. Prior to the USA's meeting with Angola in Barcelona, he was asked what he knew about the upcoming opponent. The answer was vintage Barkley. "I don't know much about Angola," he said, "but I know they're in trouble." Every NBA beat writer or sports columnist knew the following: Need a quote? Go to Charles. Need a laugh? Go to Charles. Need an athlete's opinion on a social topic? Go to Charles. Need to know the point spread in an upcoming NFL game? Go to Charles. So in 2000, the NBA's go-to guy had everybody wondering where he would go if indeed television was his next stop. He indicated to NBC that it looked like he would in fact sign with them, but after meeting with executives of Turner Broadcasting, he began to have a change of heart. He would say later that the show he watched on TNT simply looked like more fun than what he would be stepping into at NBC, and he wanted to be a part of it. Lucky us.

Charles immediately changed the landscape of sports television, not by creating some on-air persona but just by being himself. Prior to our first halftime show of the 2000–2001 season, about forty-five seconds before he and Kenny and I were going on the air live, I mentioned the first topic we'd cover. Charles looked at the Jet and asked innocently enough, "What are you gonna say?" Kenny's response: "You'll find out." And that set the tone for our show for the next fifteen seasons and counting.

If the viewers at home wondered what was going to happen next, they weren't alone. I felt the same way. Sure, we covered the NBA, but under Tim Kiely's leadership, we were allowed to stray wherever we wanted. For instance, regular on-air weigh-ins. Charles had put on some serious post-retirement pounds and had vowed to get under three hundred pounds. We had a scale in the studio so we could check his progress. Charles's willingness to step on a scale on a regular basis spoke volumes about his willingness to simply be himself and to do something that would make the show better. There was never a hint of his thinking, "Hey, this might be embarrassing. I'm a future Hall of Famer. That's off-limits!" Never happened.

And oh, by the way, as that ongoing skit reached its conclusion, we invited a professional boxer well versed in the art of the weigh-in to take part in what we hoped would be the night Charles finally made it under three hundred. Vernon Forrest was a champion in two weight classes. He was from Augusta, Georgia, and his success in the ring brought with it a huge local following in the state. Sadly, several years later he would be murdered in a late-night Atlanta robbery. But on the night that Charles shed his shirt and stepped on the scale inside our Atlanta studio, Vernon was just one of the guys celebrating with Kenny and me as Charles weighed in at 297. He had done it, never shied away from it, and it was just a taste of what the coming years would bring.

Since the only thing lacking from Charles's all-world résumé was an NBA Championship, we turned the halftime studio into something called "The Champions Club" one night. Kenny could certainly gain entrance with his two rings, and so could our guest that night, Earvin "Magic" Johnson, who had five titles. We had bouncers stationed outside the studio door next to a red carpet and velvet ropes. Magic was waved in, and he told the bouncers I was with him, so I got in, and then Kenny and Charles walked up. Kenny strolled inside while Charles stared at "The Champions Club" sign fashioned by our studio production crew. "So y'all are playing a trick on the Chuckster," he howled. During the show, Kenny, Magic, and I took turns opening the door to the studio, where strobes were flashing and techno dance music was pulsating, informing Charles that some lesser-known players who had championship rings were sending their regards. "Hey, Chuck.

Mike Penberthy sends his best. . . . Žan Tabak is dancin' in here. . . . Jack Haley says hi, and no, you can't come in." It was all live, unrehearsed, unscripted. And oh, was it a blast.

Kenny was absent from a couple shows in 2006 to be with his wife, Gwendolyn, for the birth of their child. When he returned, Charles immediately started in on our buddy, questioning why he had needed to be in California while we were working in Atlanta. Included in Kenny's explanation was the fact that he had been there to help change diapers. "I'll bet you didn't change one diaper," Charles asserted, while Kenny assured him he'd become quite proficient at the task.

It's important to point out at this juncture that on show nights there is a production meeting three hours before we go on the air. In a room adjacent to the studio, fifteen to twenty of us gather: producer, director, graphics coordinators, highlight supervisors, researchers, and me, the host of the show, whose job is to generate the discussions we have and steer the show from point A to point B. Charles, Kenny, and more recently, Shaquille O'Neal, who joined the show in 2012 after a stellar career, do not attend these meetings. The reason is twofold. We don't want those three to know what we might have up our collective sleeve on any given night. We want their reactions to whatever might happen on the show to be genuine. We also know they have no interest in being at the studio three hours early. But even though we have these meetings, sometimes the show takes an even more unexpected turn. I point this out so that you'll know nothing was discussed in the production meeting that day about diaper changing.

When Charles brought it up in the pregame show, the gears started grinding in the minds of our production crew. The decision: Charles and Kenny didn't know it, but there would be a diaper-changing contest at the end of the night. Staff runners who might normally be sent out for food or a Starbucks order were now headed to the closest shopping center to buy baby dolls and diapers. Our basketball show that night concluded at 2:00 a.m. with Charles and Kenny racing the clock to see who could change a diaper faster. For the record, Kenny proved to be quicker and much more efficient. Clearly, he had been doing this in real life in recent weeks. Charles never quite recovered from the fact that the studio camera crew, in an attempt to make things as real as possible, had melted a chocolate candy bar into the diaper that needed changing on his doll. He literally nearly hit the floor, admitting later that the sight had almost made him faint. Basketball show indeed.

Got time for another one? Good. Kobe Bryant introduced to the world the latest model in his signature line of shoes—something Nike called the Hyperdunk. And he did it with a video shot in Los Angeles in which he "jumped" over an Aston Martin apparently speeding straight at him. Kobe left his feet, the sports car flashed into and out of the frame in a blink, and Kobe landed celebrating. Well, Kenny wanted to duplicate that bit of video magic in the parking lot just outside our studio a couple hours before airtime. All he had to do was put on his new sneakers, run to a predetermined mark on the pavement, wait two seconds, and then jump like Kobe had. The production crew would do the rest. They would handle adding a car to the shot, but I had an idea that would make things a little more complicated.

Kenny went back inside to get dressed for the show while director Steve Fiorello and I had a talk. I suggested that while Kenny simply wanted to duplicate Kobe's trick, which is what he expected to see on the air later that night, it would be funnier if the car actually ran him over before he was able to leave his feet. I volunteered to be the driver. That was easy enough to shoot—a wide shot of the car entering and leaving the frame and a tight shot of me behind the wheel. But how would the car actually "hit" Kenny? I had no idea . . . but Steve did. He summoned a runner to go out and buy a blow-up doll. Yeah, you heard that right.

Well, there just so happens to be what I'll call an "adult novelty" store a mile or two from the studio, and as the story goes, the conversation inside the store went something like this:

Clerk: How can I help you?

Runner: I need a life-size blow-up doll.

Clerk: Well, we have a couple different models.

Runner: I'll take whatever is cheapest.

Oh, the glamorous life of a network runner.

What transpired in the parking lot upon his return was this. The now-inflated doll was positioned where Kenny had stood. A member of the production crew drove the car into the doll and sent it airborne. Then it was up to the director to piece all the elements together. The editing process would take most of the night, but the finished product would be ready for our postgame show. And wouldn't you know it— Kobe's Lakers had a play-off game on TNT that night. He had a huge role in LA's win and joined us live on the postgame show. This was perfect. Not only could we talk about his monster game, but Kobe and everybody else would also see for the first time Kenny's attempt to duplicate the car jump.

I can still hear the howls of laughter as if this stunt had just happened. Kenny runs to the spot . . . the car speeds into the frame . . . Kenny's image, superimposed over the soon-to-be deflated blow-up doll, is knocked out of the frame . . . and all that's left in the parking lot is a pair of shoes. Cut back to Kobe live in LA—roaring. Cut back to the videotape. I'm behind the wheel. I love my job.

What's made it work for so long is that none of us take ourselves too seriously. We're all able to laugh at ourselves. Charles can take shots at me for being the only one on the set who didn't play in the NBA, that I'm a nerd hooked on stats, that the only reason I'm on the show is that they needed a "token white guy." We can shame Charles into stepping on a scale and kid him about never winning a championship. We can jab Kenny about winning two championship rings because the legendary Hakeem "The Dream" Olajuwon carried his team to two titles. We can remind Shaq time after time after time about his struggles at the free throw line.

The guy who has steered this ship for more than twenty years is Tim Kiely, or simply TK, as he's known to everyone in the Turner hallways, who for the record is the best TV producer known to man. His feel for a show and his sense of the moment are unmatched. He knows when a discussion has run its course and will tell me in my earpiece, "Enough of this. Let's move on." He's the guy in charge of the show, but he isn't so carried away with his position that it keeps him from encouraging every person on the crew to contribute ideas that will make the show better. It is his leadership that took *Inside the NBA* to Emmy-winning levels several times over and made every man and woman on our crew feel important to the show's success.

In our first year working together in the mid-1990s, TK had just come to Turner from ESPN, where the philosophy was to make the highlights of games in progress as up-to-date as possible. Sometimes that meant the studio host would have to voice a highlight without having seen it. Up to that point in my studio shows at TNT, the preferred course was to show me a highlight off air first, and then I'd do it live. TK was trying to change that, and I was going to have to adjust. We had gone through a pretty rocky postgame show one night, with a lot of late highlights added that I hadn't seen. It wasn't my best night. Afterward, we had a conversation in the control room, which continued into the hallway, which made its way into the men's room, where I was rinsing out my coffee mug, and things were getting heated. How heated? Well, let's just say I took my freshly rinsed coffee mug and fired it against the wall. As it shattered into a zillion ceramic pieces, I brushed by TK on my way out the door, put my game notes from that night in my office, and hit the road.

The next day I went to the studio for another show, and as I walked into my office, I noticed a box on my desk. Inside was a new coffee mug. It was white with a newspaper want ad emblazoned on it: "Postal Worker Wanted." Yep, I had crossed the line the night before. I found TK in his office and apologized for being unprofessional, for being stubborn and resistant to change. I promised to adapt, realizing that his methods were not designed to prove his authority but simply to make me a better host and in turn to make the show better. These days we still laugh at that night and that mug, which still sits on a shelf in my office. It's a constant reminder that the show we do is not about me; it's about everybody on the crew who shows up night in and night out and busts their butts to make the show what it is. And what it is, in my mind, is a distraction from all the real-life stuff we're bombarded with from the internet and the daily news. There are days it seems the earth has spun off its axis. You're afraid to watch the network news some nights because things have gotten more and more out of control. But you know that later that night you can turn on "that basketball show" on TNT, escape for a few hours, and laugh.

You know who watches the show every night? My eighty-six-year-old mother, Lois. In fact, she's watched me on TV whenever possible since she was my forty-eight-year-old mother and I was just getting my start in Macon. I'm floored by her devotion, constant encouragement, and attention to detail. Back when I was anchoring the weekend sports at WSB-TV in Atlanta, it was not uncommon for me to get a phone call or have a face-to-face conversation with her that went something like this:

"Ernie, we watched your 6:00 report on Saturday night, and it was *so* good."

"Thanks, Mom. That's exactly what I expect to hear from my mom."

"But your dad and I agree you looked like you either hadn't put on any makeup or hadn't shaved, and you really need to pay attention to that."

"Thanks, Mom."

The thing is she was right. I was so busy on those Saturday and Sunday nights, and WSB wasn't providing a makeup artist in those days, so yeah, there were nights I went on the air with a visible five-o'clock shadow. But from that point on, I made sure I looked my best.

My mother is beautiful. Guys talk about marrying over their heads or, in a football analogy, "outkicking their coverage." No doubt I did when I married Cheryl, and my father certainly did when he married Lois Denhard. She is a vibrant, piano-playing, gourmet-cooking, family-loving treasure who held us together while married to a husband whose job kept him away from home for long periods of time during every baseball season.

She had a magnet stuck to the refrigerator that proclaimed, "We now interrupt this marriage to bring you the baseball season." She was the glue that held our family together. Folks who meet my mother for the first time always come away with the same impression—incredibly sharp, with boundless energy, an infectious laugh, and charm. They liken her to Betty White, who with advancing age has become more popular than ever, and I certainly see the resemblance. But Lois Johnson is Betty White on steroids. My dad used to say that Mom was "tougher than a two-dollar steak." We watched her rebound from horrible bouts with asthma throughout her life and then give cancer a swift kick in the backside, not once but twice. If there's ever been a better snapshot of grace, elegance, humor, and world-class toughness, I haven't seen it.

And I never will.

7

Unforgettable Moments

WHILE BASKETBALL HAS BEEN AT THE CENTER of my workload at TNT, it is far from the only assignment I've been given in my twenty-eight years there. I've done play-by-play, worked the sidelines, and hosted the studio for Major League Baseball, the NFL, golf, Wimbledon tennis, track and field, boxing, rowing, Olympic speed skating, team handball, weight lifting, judo, modern pentathlon (horses and riders going through various disciplines), and even a motorcycle jump by Robbie Knievel on an aircraft carrier docked in New York. This job has allowed me to see the world—Cuba, France, Norway, England, Scotland, Russia, South Africa, and Australia. And with such vast opportunities, I've acquired a lifetime of memories when the unscripted became reality.

Dan Jansen's Olympic odyssey certainly qualifies. He was arguably the world's best speed skater in 1988 when the games were held in Calgary, Alberta, Canada. Before skating in the 500-meter sprint, in which he was favored to win gold, he learned that his sister Jane had lost her battle with leukemia. That day he raced and fell in the first turn. Four days later in the 1,000 meters, on world-record pace, he fell again. This was unheard of. Ask anyone close to the sport and they will tell you these world-class athletes stay on skates as easily as you and I stay on our feet while walking around the mall. The tragic loss of his sister, combined with the crushing result on the ice, made Dan Jansen a sympathetic figure in America during those '88 games.

He would have another chance four years later in Albertville, France. The heartbreak of 1988 replayed on TV screens around the world before he competed. But again he came away empty-handed, leaving France without a medal. The year 1994 would be the last chance for this national champion to finally show his best on the Olympic stage. I had called his 1992 races on TNT and now found myself in Hamar, Norway, at a spectacular venue known as the Viking Ship—it resembled the upside-down keel of a ship—and it was packed every day with perhaps the most knowledgeable speed-skating fans on the planet. Norwegians know the sport, study the split times, and can recite world records the way Americans can rattle off baseball stats and records.

Ten thousand people inside the Viking Ship all knew Dan Jansen's story. And they could feel his disappointment when he finished out of the medals in the 500 meters. That just made his performance in the 1,000 meters even more special. In his last chance at Olympic glory, he came up golden, and he did it in world-record time. It was a breathtaking moment to be at the microphone. But it paled in comparison to what happened next. He skated a victory lap holding his daughter, named Jane, in his late sister's honor, while a standing-room-only crowd cheered and waved and cried. Blackberries don't come much sweeter than that.

Covering golf's Open Championship, or the British Open, if you will, has taken me to the birthplace of the game—St. Andrews in Scotland. What I witnessed and described on TNT in 2005 will stick with me forever. Jack Nicklaus was putting the finishing touches on his legendary career. As the all-time leader with eighteen professional major championships, he was playing in his final major, and it was at this historic site. He was sixty-five years old, and while no one harbored the illusion he would win the Claret Jug for the fourth time, everybody was hoping he might summon all of his one-of-a-kind skills and championship pedigree to make the Friday cut and play the weekend. What a Sunday send-off he would get from the Scottish gallery.

In the late stages of round two on Friday, it became apparent that would not happen—too much ground to make up and not enough time. Everybody knew it. And so everybody, and I mean all of Scotland, started converging outside the eighteenth fairway and green as the Golden Bear made his way toward the finishing hole. Calling Jack's final hole in major competition was easy. For 90 percent of the time, I just shut up. The pictures told the story. There was the tee shot down the middle; the long photo opportunity as he crossed the famed landmark, the Swilken Bridge, where he stood and savored the moment; the approach that ran past the hole; and the left-to-right perfectly paced putt that found the bottom of the cup for a birdie. The roars were deafening. The emotions were pure. The adulation was overwhelming. There was, as I said on the air that day, "not a dry eye in the country." What an honor to be there.

The Jansen gold and the Golden Bear's stirring farewell to the Old Course were two sporting moments that make me appreciate the opportunity to do this job for a living. They were both unforgettable. So was my flight home from Brisbane, Australia, after the Goodwill Games of 2001, but the circumstances were far different. It came on America's darkest day. Our TNT crew had been in Australia for more than three weeks, and I was anchoring our daily coverage of that multisport, Olympic-style competition. Our set was located on a man-made beach just outside the city, and we had a blast. I worked barefoot most of the time; athletes would come on for interviews; I took a kangaroo for a walk on the beach, held a koala bear, which didn't smell very good and had very sharp claws, and played a drum with some aboriginal musicians. We did that kind of stuff while at the same time showing two weeks of competition. As much fun as we all had, we couldn't wait to get back to the States. We were scheduled to land in Los Angeles, then fly to Atlanta.

The date was September 11, 2001.

The wheels touched down at LAX around 10:30 a.m. As we taxied to the terminal, we heard the captain on his microphone. "Folks, we have landed in Los Angeles, and you might notice out your windows that there's not much activity. Without getting into any detail, I can tell you that there has been a national emergency, and every airport in the country has been shut down. The only reason we were even allowed to land here is that we did not have enough fuel to reroute. When we get to the gate, please gather your belongings and make your way inside. Law enforcement officers will tell you what to do next."

There was no panic on board, just quizzical looks, until one of our senior producers, Howard Zalkowitz, sitting two rows in front of me, placed a quick phone call and delivered the news. "Planes hit the twin towers in New York. They're both down. Another plane crashed into the Pentagon." I borrowed his phone and called home. My oldest daughter, Maggie, fourteen, had been in school when it had all happened. "Dad! Are you all right? I saw the planes on TV. It's awful, and I knew you were on a plane. When are you coming home?" At that point, I really didn't have an answer to that last question.

We were met by FBI agents at the gate and escorted to baggage claim, where we gathered our luggage and were told that buses would pick us up and take us to the nearby rental car area, where we would be taken to a hotel. We would stay there until airline travel was permitted again, and no one knew when that might be—hours? days? Nobody knew. But I knew this. I was going home. Now. That was a feeling shared by our director, Steve Fiorello, and one of our videotape operators, Mike Winslow. We had families who had circled this date—the end of that long Australia adventure—and we had talked to our loved ones and heard the anguish. So we rented a van, and at 1:00 LA time, about seven hours after this 9/11 nightmare had started, we set out on a cross-country drive to Atlanta.

The three of us drove in three-hour shifts, with the radio tuned to the nonstop coverage of what had gone on in New York, Washington, and Shanksville, Pennsylvania. When we weren't in the driver's seat, we tried to get a little sleep, called home to assure our wives we were doing okay, or rode shotgun with a road map, seeking the best way home.

When we stopped, it was quick. Fill up the gas tank, get some food to go, keep movin'. It was a twenty-two-hundred-mile trip. A couple things stood out as we drove late that September 11 night through New Mexico. It was such a crystal clear night that when I woke from a nap in the backseat, the first thing I saw were stars that seemed so close you could reach out and touch them. And at one point we got to a spot so remote that when we hit the search button on the radio to try to get a station, it cycled through the entire band without stopping. Silver City, New Mexico, will always have a special place in my heart. In danger of running out of gas, we were able to fill up there at 2:00 a.m.

The next morning we stopped for coffee and more gas and realized we weren't the only ones traversing the country. Four sailors in uniform were driving from San Diego to the East Coast and were refilling their tank. Hitting Interstate 20 in Texas was our short-term goal. Once we got on that, we could ride it straight into downtown Atlanta, but that drive through Texas and Louisiana and Mississippi and Alabama seemed interminable. There was little talking, lots of snoring, and all kinds of time to think.

As I thought about the flight from Australia, I was struck by the timing of a request I had made to a flight attendant early that Tuesday morning. I had awoken to see the most amazing sunrise out my window. Layers upon layers of brilliant colors stacked on top of each other. Back then it wasn't totally uncommon for a passenger to ask if maybe for just a minute the pilot would allow him a look from the cockpit. I had asked the flight attendant if that was possible, given how brilliant the sunrise was, and she had said, "Sure, let me check and see." She had returned a few minutes later and said she was sorry, but they were pretty busy. I started doing the math in my head as I rode in the backseat. I realized I had made that request to go to the cockpit when all hell was breaking loose in the skies over the United States.

Thirty-five hours after leaving Los Angeles on Tuesday afternoon, 9/11, we pulled into the parking lot of Turner Broadcasting at 3:00 a.m. on Thursday. Steve, Mike, and I got into our own cars and drove to our own homes. I walked into the house at 4:00 a.m. and turned on the TV. I had not yet seen one second of what had happened on Tuesday. It didn't take long for the images to be broadcast again. I had heard all the descriptions on the radio during our cross-country drive. Now I was seeing the footage, and the destruction, and the looks of sheer desperation on the faces of New Yorkers wondering if their loved ones had somehow survived. I walked into the bedroom and gave my sleeping wife a kiss on the cheek and told her not to get up. I was just going to stay up, sit in the den, and be the first thing my kids saw when they came downstairs that morning.

———————————

I wrote a poem about 9/11. You'd never know that unless you were a member of the Turner Sports staff or one of the handful of TV guys from the NBA who were gathered in a hotel conference room for the annual seminar previewing the upcoming 2001–2002 season.

A little background. For years now, I've written poetry for fun. Once I heard Pete Van Wieren, one of my dad's old broadcast partners, deliver at a banquet a poem he had written. It was touching and funny, and I admired Pete's ability to do that. Later I learned that the legendary coach John

Wooden wrote poetry to keep his mind sharp. So around 1995, I decided I was going to try to write a poem and read it at our end of the NFL season wrap party. It told the story of our eight weeks of traveling from city to city, and I weaved in tales that involved our crew members, some of which they would prefer not to have repeated in public. Before I knew it, I had a couple pages, and while the rhymes were often pretty juvenile, it was a hit! People laughed. They applauded. They wanted copies. They wanted me to read it again. Amazing the effect bad poetry can have on people.

Over the next twenty years, I wrote poems for annual Turner meetings before the NBA or MLB seasons. I wrote them for individuals like Alonzo Mourning and Dominique Wilkins and John Wooden and Charles Barkley and read them at banquets where they were being honored. I still write and recite a new one every year for the NBA's Legends Brunch during All-Star Weekend. I've been asked to write them for Turner employees who are retiring or moving on to other jobs. In 2014, as Turner Sports was negotiating with the NBA to remain a broadcast partner, my boss Lenny Daniels asked me to write a poem that I would deliver to fewer than twenty people. Six were NBA owners—the guys we had to convince that the league needed TNT. I have no idea if I helped our cause, but we got the contract. And weeks later, as the *Sports Business Journal* chronicled what is always a lengthy and tense negotiation process, I was stunned to read this:

> In Atlanta the league's media committees toured Turner's NBA studios, meeting with top Turner executives. An unlikely effective moment came during a general session meeting when Turner NBA broadcaster Ernie Johnson came into the

meeting and recited a 20-paragraph poem rhyming the network's commitment to the NBA. The lighthearted verse was meant to entertain, but also show how much Turner valued its relationship with the league. The two have been partners for the better part of three decades. "It was goose-bump fantastic," said Washington Wizards owner Ted Leonsis, who chaired the owners media committee. "It was one of those little things that showed the right touch, and reconfirmed that they were a great partner."[1]

Well, that was just about the nicest thing anybody's ever said about my poetry. I do it for fun, but I've found that for just a few minutes it brings a group together. We laugh at ourselves and each other, and that's never a bad thing.

In 2001, I didn't know if I wanted to write a poem for the preseason NBA seminar. It had been just a little over a month since the 9/11 attacks. If I did compose something, should I just keep it to basketball and what had gone on in the off-season? So yes, I did write one. And no, it wasn't just about basketball.

On That September Tuesday

It happens every mid-July, the cycle starts anew.
Guys get signed or they get traded. Let's highlight a
few.
Patrick Ewing's on the move. He's found a brand-
new home.
He's in the Sunshine State, where lots of other seniors
roam.

The Nets and Suns pulled off a trade with Stephon
dealt for Kidd.
Tim Hardaway's in Dallas now, just one thing Cuban
did.

Avery Johnson went to Denver. LA is Richmond's
team.
The Hawks got better quickly with Shareef
Abdur-Rahim.

Derek Anderson's in Portland now. Steve Smith's in
San Antone.
Houston hopes Glen Rice's "J" will bust up every
zone.
And remember how Chris Webber looked when Sac-
ramento lost?
The Kings resigned their heart and soul, no matter
what it cost.

It hardly made the headlines, not even in Detroit.
Brian Cardinal's not a star, though he is fairly adroit.
But check the league transaction list, some of you
may remember.
He signed his Piston contract on the tenth day of
September.

On that September Monday, we thought, "Hey, is
this the week?"
Michael's got his mind made up, so when's he gonna
speak?
And suddenly the prospect of his imminent return
Was jolted from our minds as we watched two cities
burn.

On that September Tuesday, well, our view forever
changed.
We paid no mind to matters like those schedules
we'd arranged.
Our eyes transfixed on images that chilled our very
souls

And shook us at the cornerstone of all our dreams
and goals.

On that September Tuesday, we just watched in
disbelief,
Security and innocence the targets of a thief
Who sees the loss of life from some altered state of
mind.
Evil showed its face that day in horror undefined.

On that September Tuesday, it seems we made a
pact.
We'll send the world a message from this land that
was attacked.
Stories of the people who responded at Ground
Zero
Gave us all a brand-new way to recognize a hero.

On that September Tuesday, there was courage in
those rows
Of passengers who took a stand. Yes, let's remember
those.
And all who reached a hand to help in any way they
could,
From the streets of New York City to your own
neighborhood.

On that September Tuesday, the Father heard our
pleas.
And in the days to follow you could find us on our
knees.
We seek his comfort, seek his face, seek his almighty
power.
For Scripture tells us that the Lord above is our
strong tower.

On that September Tuesday, we were jolted wide
    awake.
To the man or group responsible, you've made a big
    mistake.
This nation, it is resolute. It defends and yes it fights.
Look no farther than this park, for here Atlanta
    unites.

On that September Tuesday, we were moved so many
    ways.
Sad and angry, violated—it's been that way for days.
But mixed in with the hurt and the tears that won't
    run dry
Is the knowledge that Americans can hear this coun-
    try cry.

So on this October Wednesday, with the season al-
    most here,
We know that many folks out there can't shake this
    haunting fear.
And now perhaps they look to us, much more than
    years before,
As simply a departure as this country wages war.

It's a challenge we can't sidestep, and in fact we
    should embrace it.
There's not a better bunch to take this on, come on
    let's face it.
And so we start a season that will be unlike the rest,
And under the conditions, let's make sure we give
    our best.

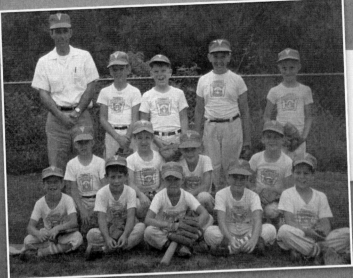

The Vees, authors of the original blackberry moment. I'm the scrawny kid second from the right, middle row.

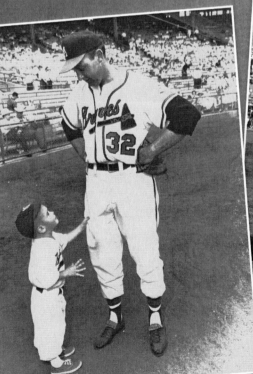

My father, Ernie Johnson Sr., the man I always looked up to.

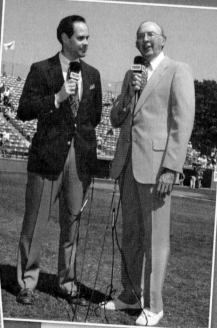

The highlight of my career. Working with Dad in the midnineties.

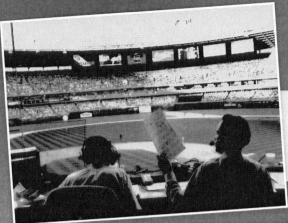

When you're working with your dad, it's the best seat in the house.

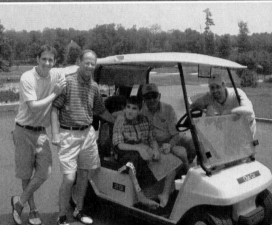

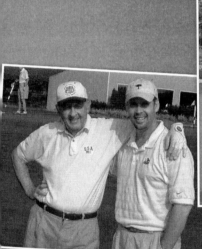

With Dad, Eric, Michael, and brother-in-law Jacky, ready for another round in what we called "The Johnson Open."

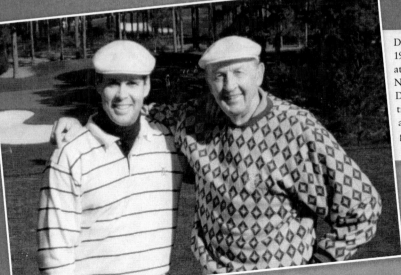

December 10, 1998. A round at Augusta National with Dad, the one time I wanted a round of golf to go slower.

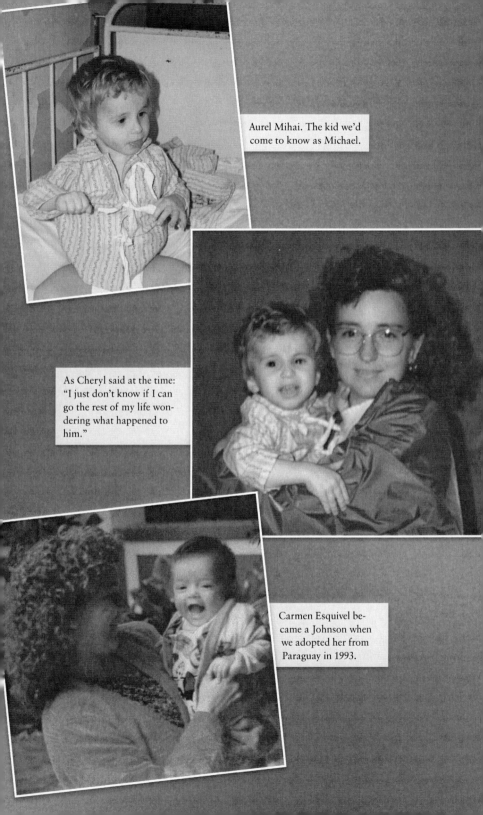

Aurel Mihai. The kid we'd come to know as Michael.

As Cheryl said at the time: "I just don't know if I can go the rest of my life wondering what happened to him."

Carmen Esquivel became a Johnson when we adopted her from Paraguay in 1993.

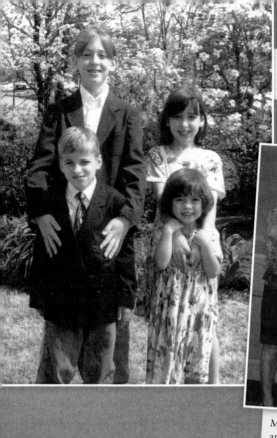

Eric, Maggie, Michael, and Carmen. We thought this was it as far as kids go. We were wrong.

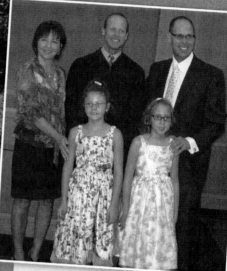

Meet the newest Johnson girls, Allison and Ashley, adopted out of foster care in 2011.

Eric had us outfitted in T-shirts he designed to celebrate the adoption of Allison and

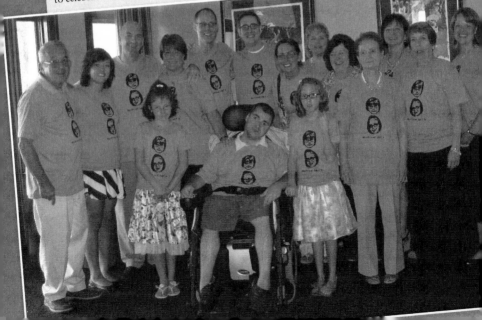

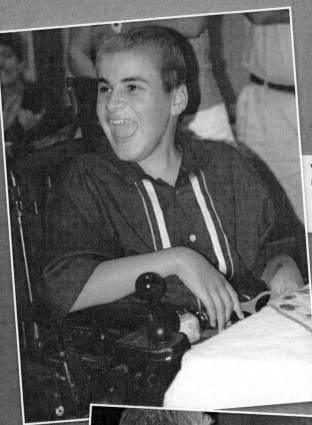

Why is Michael smiling? He got a new lawn mower he could watch me use for his birthday. I'm serious.

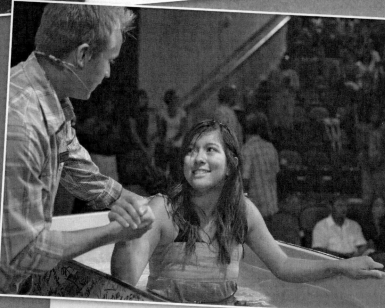

That unscripted moment when Carmen surprised us by going forward to be baptized at 12Stone Church.

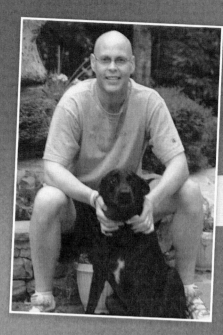

Chemo, 2006. "You may have cancer, but it doesn't have you."

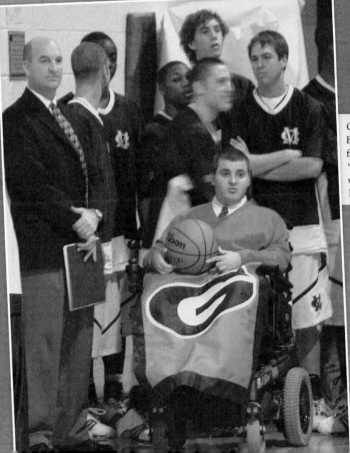

Coach Phil Bollier with his five-foot-tall "impact player with no vertical leap."

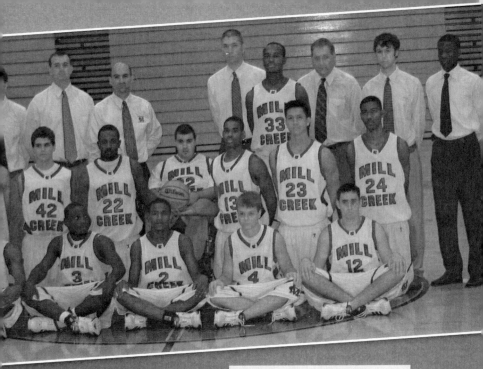

Picture day with the Mill Creek Hawks.

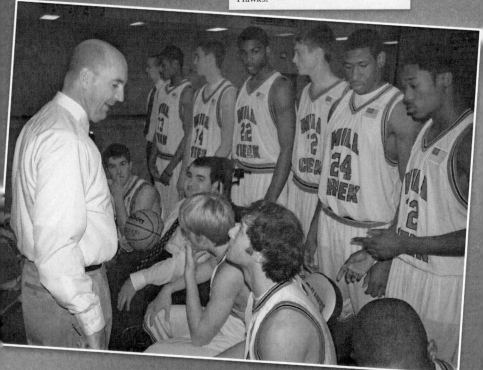

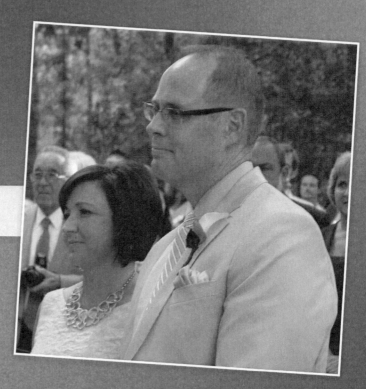

The love
of my life,
Cheryl.

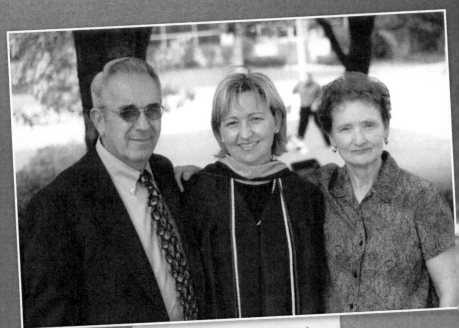

Cheryl with her mom and dad, Lou and
Joan, after earning her master's degree in
2001.

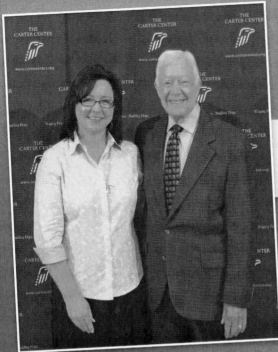

Cheryl with former president Jimmy Carter after she spoke on the issue of child sex trafficking at the Mobilizing Faith for Women Forum.

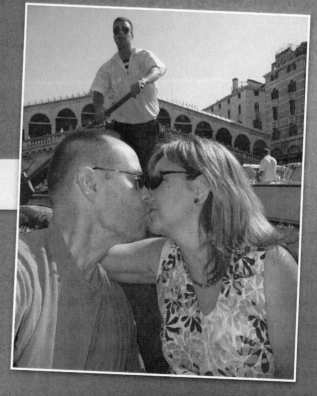

I'll never forget our twenty-fifth anniversary trip to Italy.

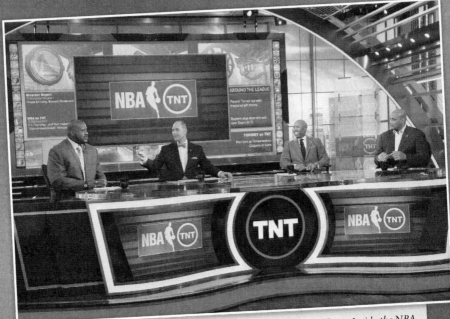

Shaq, Kenny, and Charles. I never had brothers growing up, but I do on *Inside the* NBA.

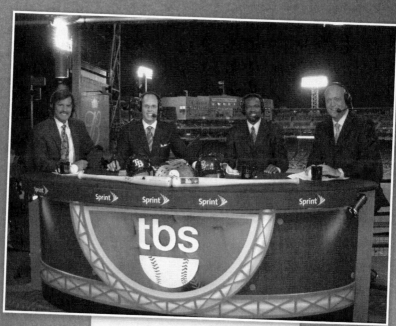

On the TBS MLB Playoff set with Dennis Eckersly, Harold Reynolds, and Cal Ripken Jr.

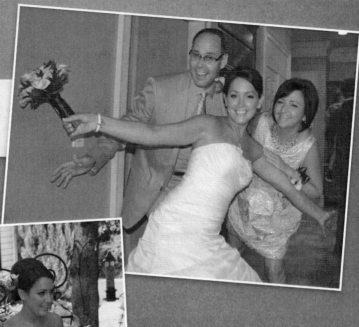

Maggie's wedding day in 2012. One of my all-time favorite shots.

Walking Maggie down the aisle. Terrifying and exhilarating all at once.

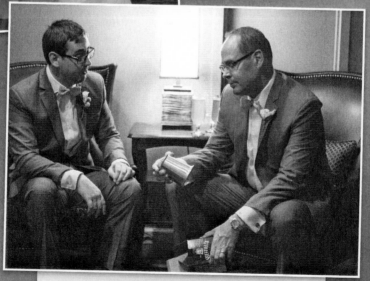

Eric presents me with a mug engraved with "My Best Man, My Best Friend," just as I had done with my father thirty years earlier.

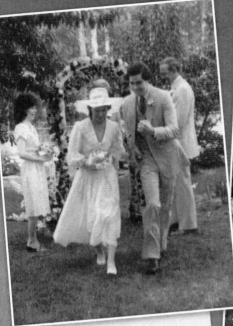

It was an unscripted fist pump when Cheryl and I were married in 1982.

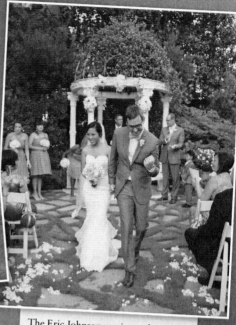

The Eric Johnson version as he and Quynh became man and wife in 2012.

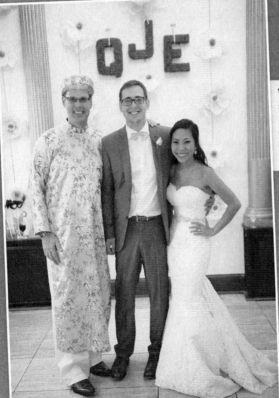

Wearing the traditional Vietnamese "áo-dài" for Eric and Quynh's second wedding ceremony in two days.

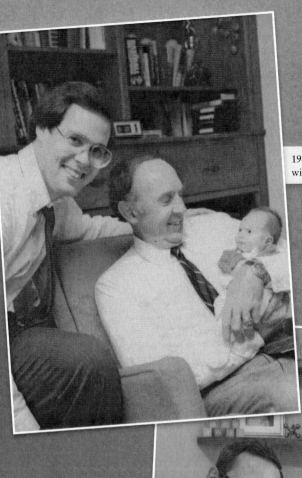

1984. My dad and me with my firstborn, Eric.

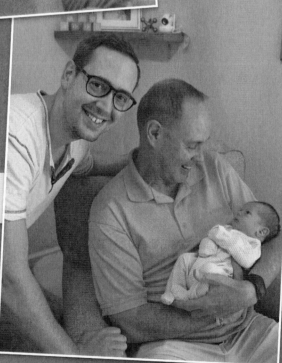

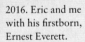

2016. Eric and me with his firstborn, Ernest Everett.

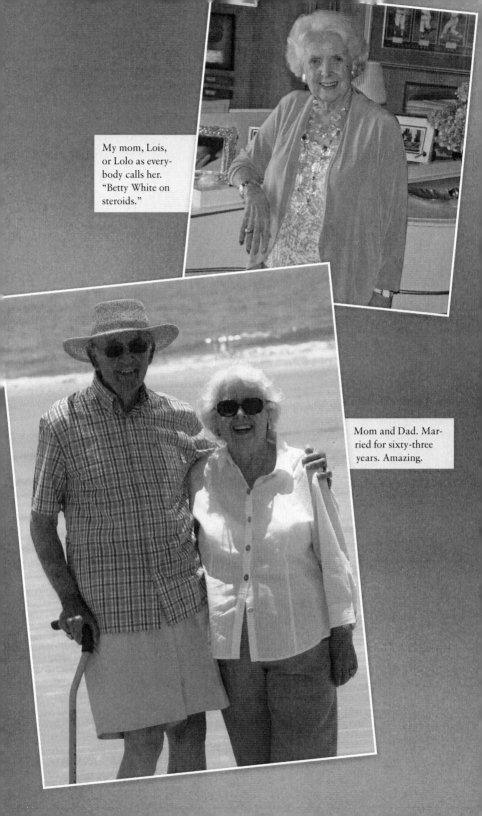

My mom, Lois, or Lolo as everybody calls her. "Betty White on steroids."

Mom and Dad. Married for sixty-three years. Amazing.

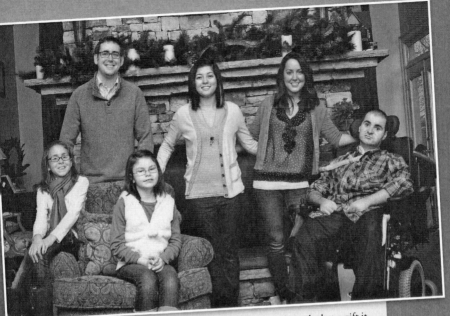

This photograph was a Christmas gift from the kids, and what a gift it was!

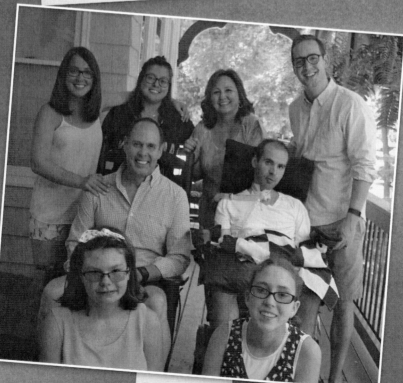

Father's Day, 2016.

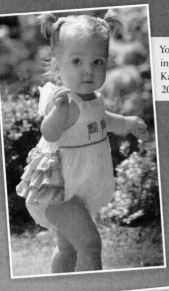

You've probably heard it before. Having grandchildren is off the charts. Katie Ann Pruitt in the spring of 2016.

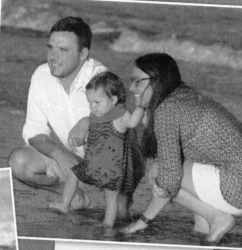

There is nothing quite like seeing your kids become parents. Maggie and Dustin with Katie Ann.

Eric and Quynh with Ernest Everett.

Poppy and Nonna with Everett and Katie.

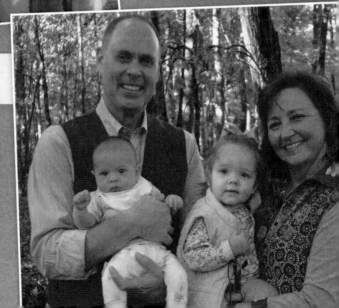

8

Bump

THE YEAR 2003 was going to be a great year for Turner Sports for a couple reasons. In February, TNT would for the first time televise the NBA All-Star Game. We'd been a part of that weekend for ages, the highlight for us being All-Star Saturday Night with the slam dunk contest and the three-point shoot-out. But as much fun as those events were, there was always a kind of empty feeling because by the time the game itself was played, our coverage had already ended. I'd be on the first plane out on Sunday morning, later watching the game at home. But after the new television contracts were hammered out, two of the major changes had Turner now owning All-Star Weekend, including the game, and ESPN now broadcasting the NBA draft, which we had done for years. I loved the trade-off.

The other biggie was that in July we would now have a share of the British Open, or as they call it in the United Kingdom, the Open Championship. I've always loved the game of golf and was thrilled in 1995 when executive producer Mike Pearl called me into his office and told me I would have a role in Turner's coverage of the PGA Championship at Riviera in Los Angeles. That was a new responsibility for me, and to say that I had questions about doing golf play-by-play, or hole-by-hole, as it's called, would be a massive understatement. A few years earlier, Jim Nantz of CBS, whose expertise has had him at the microphone for just about every major event on the American sports landscape, was visiting Atlanta on a night when I was working the NBA studio. During a few free minutes before the crew prepared for a halftime show, Jim and I had a chance to chat, and as we were talking, he said out of the blue, "You've got a good voice for golf. You should consider that." I thanked him for the compliment but never thought it would happen. Now it was about to.

As it turns out, the basic format of the coverage was pretty simple. Our partnership with CBS for the PGA Championship was already well established before I assumed my role in 1995, so I stepped into a system that was already well oiled. Turner would have the Thursday and Friday coverage, about six hours a day, and then three hours of early coverage on the weekend mornings before CBS took over for the rest of the day. The CBS announcing crew had their tower, and we at Turner had ours overlooking the eighteenth green. Analysts on the ground were walking with select groups, and basically, CBS had the odd-numbered holes and Turner had the evens. I just listened to the producer in my headset, in this case the legendary Frank Chirkinian or, when he stepped away for a break on those long days, Lance Barrow, who would eventually succeed Frank and remains in the CBS producer's chair to this day. And on those weekend mornings, David Winner would take the controls. The producer would identify the hole we were going to and the golfer we'd see, and if it was an even-numbered hole, I would talk. But there were certain rules to follow, and I got a briefing on these from Verne Lundquist in the days leading up to round one.

Verne is as talented a broadcaster as has ever put on a headset, and he is as gracious a gentleman as you'll find.

"What can you tell me about what I can expect this week?" I asked. Verne's words have stuck with me to this day.

"Just remember you're a caption writer. Less is often more. Folks are watching their televisions. You write the caption for what you just saw. If you are going to tell a story that adds to what viewers are seeing, make sure it's quick, because we'll be showing a lot of golf shots and moving from hole to hole quickly. Don't get caught in the middle of a long story when you're told to throw it to another hole. Don't worry. You'll get a feel for the rhythm."

I was a six-foot-three sponge as we sat in a golf cart in the massive TV compound, Verne speaking and me listening.

"Oh, and there's another thing you must remember. Frank hates it when an announcer speaks when a player is making contact, so let that moment live on its own. We want to hear the impact."

On Thursday, as Verne took a thirty-minute break about three hours deep into our coverage of the first round, I put on the headset and waited for the first even-numbered hole cue from the production truck. Remember that advice I'd gotten from Verne? The first few times I did exactly what he'd told me, and he was right. I was getting a feel for the rhythm and was feeling so comfortable that in no time at all I was breaking all the rules—talking over tee shots just as club face was meeting golf ball and painting myself into a corner by starting a story about something I'd learned about Riviera while walking the course on Tuesday and Wednesday with no chance of finishing the story before I was told to send it to another hole. It certainly hadn't escaped Frank Chirkinian, whose voice soon filled my headset with the not-so-gentle reminder that we never (translated *never*!) talk while the golf ball is being struck and that it would be a good idea for me to toss coverage to the next hole when I'm told and not when I want to.

After that thirty-minute baptism into the world of televised golf, even with the mistakes, I left the golf course with a feeling that wasn't quite satisfaction but also with encouragement. I knew not only that I could do a better job the next day but also that I would. I had prepared, I had done my absolute best in what was a foreign broadcast setting, and I had learned valuable lessons from the very best in the business that would serve me well for the next twenty PGA Championships.

The British Open was still five months away as we prepared for our first NBA All-Star Game on TNT in February. It would be played in Atlanta, where I live, which was cool because for the first time I wouldn't have to head out of town for All-Star Weekend. It would be Michael Jordan's last All-Star Game as he played his final NBA season, so at Turner Sports we were all pretty jacked up about having it on our air. And then came one of those unscripted moments that turn into a life-changing episode.

I was shaving one morning a few days before the game and was trying to knock down a few stray whiskers above my left jawbone near my ear. Guys reading this know that when you shave, you screw up your face all different ways to make the skin taut, and when I did this, moving my mouth to the right, I noticed a bump under the skin became visible near my left ear. When I relaxed my face, it disappeared. So I repeated the move. There it was again. Trying to make sense of this and calm my nerves, I thought, "Maybe there's something near my right ear similar to the left," so I moved my mouth to the left to tighten the skin on the right side, hoping I'd see the same kind of bump. Nothing. So what now? My plan did not include going to the doctor, at least not now. It was All-Star Weekend, and we would be busy around the clock. "Besides," I thought, "maybe it's nothing to be concerned about and it'll go away on its own."

The All-Star Game of 2003 gave us all we could have hoped for in our inaugural TNT broadcast. Vince Carter gave up his starting spot to Michael Jordan in his last All-Star appearance, and when MJ hit a three-pointer in overtime to give the East a two-point lead, it looked like he might end the night holding the MVP trophy. I would be at center court for the ceremony as Commissioner David Stern handed out the hardware.

I always spend the last few minutes of an All-Star Game in a courtside seat preparing for the interview I will conduct with the MVP, and there are usually two or three guys who can get it depending on who wins, East or West. If the outcome isn't much in doubt, I pretty much have an idea who the media members will choose as they're handed slips of paper to jot down their choice. In this case, I had been preparing for the possibility of Allen Iverson, who had thirty-five points, or Tracy McGrady, who had twenty-nine. Now that Michael had hit the big three, my focus shifted to him.

But hold everything. Jermaine O'Neal was whistled for a foul as Kobe Bryant launched a three with one second left. Kobe hit two of his three free throws to tie the game, and we headed to a second overtime. Kevin Garnett scored the first seven points for the West in that second overtime period, finished with thirty-seven points, and claimed MVP honors. We did our quick two-minute interview at center court on TNT "feeding the house," as it's called when our interview is also piped through the arena's PA system, and our very first NBA All-Star Game was in the books. It was every bit as much fun as we all hoped it would be.

As the NBA's regular season resumed after the All-Star Game, so did what had now become a shaving ritual for me— always checking that "thing" by my left ear. When the NBA play-offs began in April, it was still there. It hadn't gotten any bigger; it hadn't gotten any smaller. It didn't hurt, and if you looked at me on the air or face-to-face, you couldn't see anything. But I knew it was there, and it was becoming one of those things that wouldn't leave the back of my mind. I could be having a great day off, hanging with the family, but there was this gnawing feeling that something wasn't right. And let's be perfectly honest here. I was scared, and deep down inside I don't think I wanted to know if there was a serious problem. So I continued to take the easy and stupid route. I did my best to ignore the bump and hope that one morning I would wake up and it would have mysteriously disappeared.

Every play-off season when the NBA reaches the conference finals, we take our studio show on the road. Dallas and

San Antonio would play a best of seven series in the West in 2003, and we would do our shows from those arenas. When I looked at the play-off schedule, I saw a big-time conflict. If the Mavs and the Spurs went the distance, the seventh game in San Antonio would fall on Saturday, May 31. The high school graduation of my firstborn son, Eric, was scheduled for . . . wait for it . . . Saturday, May 31.

A game seven between the Mavs and the Spurs would be our biggest TNT game of the season, and because Turner had no role in the broadcast of the NBA Finals, it would be our last telecast of the season. So how was I to handle this? It was one of those situations that parents from coast to coast have had to meet head-on. You feel like you're doing a pretty good job navigating that often tenuous highway called balancing family and work when you come to a fork in the road. Often you can determine your course without much thought, and without taking your foot off the gas, you choose your path, full speed ahead. But in this case, I had to pump the brakes, pull over to the shoulder, and stare at the signs in front of me. Game seven or graduation? Choose one.

One of the many valuable lessons I learned from my father was work ethic. Another was loyalty. Both were in play here. The only time I remember my dad missing a game as a Braves' broadcaster was when my oldest sister, Dawn, got married. Otherwise, he was there night after night behind the microphone. I'm sure there were nights it hurt him deeply to miss various events in our lives, and certainly there were times when I wished he could have been sitting in the stands at my Little League baseball game, but there was also the understanding in our house that this was simply the nature of Dad's job. It's just the way it was. He had an unwavering loyalty to his job and the organization that had given him the opportunity, and he never took it for granted. If ever there was a "company man," it was my father, and he passed that on to me. That's what made my situation so tough. I didn't want to let the company down. I didn't want to let Eric down. (Please, a show of hands if you've been there so I don't have to feel like the Lone Ranger? Good. Thank you.)

I didn't immediately tell Cheryl about the what-ifs I was wrestling with, hoping that maybe the NBA would announce a change in the schedule before the series started, but that didn't happen. "Maybe," I thought, "the graduation will be in the morning, and I can fly from Dallas to Atlanta after game six, go to graduation, and fly to San Antonio in time for game seven." Nope. Graduation was at night. So before I left for the conference finals, we sat down and talked it over, and I laid it all out. I made my decision, and she said she understood. The decision (drumroll, please) was that on Saturday, May 31, 2003, if there was a game seven in the Western Conference Finals, there was only one place I could be, and that was at the graduation ceremony for Collins Hill High School. The bottom line was this: I am a dad who happens to be a sportscaster. Not the other way around. Now would my bosses see it that way?

The first step was to tell my producer, Tim Kiely. He and his wife, Maureen, had become parents of twins a few years earlier, and so the fatherhood/work thing was not a foreign concept for him. Although a high school graduation scenario was still years away for him, he knew exactly where I was coming from, shook my hand, and said he'd get back to me as soon as he took the issue upstairs. And so I waited for the response from upper management. What if they said,

"No way!" I was envisioning a high-noon standoff with the brass—an ultimatum given to me, a resignation given to them, all over a game that might not even be played. When TK returned to my office, he said it was all taken care of. He admitted there was not 100 percent approval from all parties, but from the parties that really mattered, I had the green light to attend graduation. Anxiety gave way to relief, but to be honest, I hoped it would all be a moot point in the long run. Not that there was any doubt in my mind I was doing the right thing, but I didn't want to let down Charles and Kenny, or any of my colleagues on the crew, at the climax of our NBA run for that season.

The San Antonio Spurs appeared to be cooperating. After dropping the opener at home, they reeled off three straight wins, including two in Dallas, and Tim Duncan and company were sittin' pretty. They had a 3–1 lead and were heading back to San Antonio with a chance to close things out in five. Shoot, I'd be back home in Atlanta with a few days to spare before Eric walked at graduation. When we hit the air with *Inside the NBA* after game five in San Antonio, I said something like this: "The Dallas Mavericks are still alive in the Western Conference Finals. The final here in San Antonio is Mavs 103, Spurs 91. There will be a game six in Dallas on Thursday night." The Mavericks had played as gutsy a play-off game as you'll see. Trailing going into the fourth quarter on the road, facing elimination, they had outscored the Spurs 29–10 in the fourth quarter to extend the series. Let me be clear on something here too. In this job, we don't root for teams. If there's anything we root for, it's compelling basketball. A series sweep in any year is fun only for the team doing the sweeping. We want the kind of series that has viewers looking forward to the next pivotal game, planning to get home or go to the sports bar to watch the next chapter unfold. Certainly, we had that now after the clutch Dallas win in game five.

As we do on every game day on the road, we had a morning production meeting before game six in Dallas that night. It's an hour of eating bacon and eggs and laying out our plans for the pregame, halftime, and postgame shows. What story lines we want to explore, what video of the Dallas win in game five we want to break down on the air, that sort of thing. As things wrapped up, I felt it was appropriate to address our production crew, the men and women who cut the highlights, create the graphics, and do the research and the stats throughout the season. I simply wanted to say thanks for all the hard work and the endless hours they'd put in. If the series ended that night, there would be no other opportunity for me to do it.

And then I added the "but if" part of the equation. If the series did not end and there was a game seven, I wouldn't be in San Antonio but at my son's high school graduation. Having already received the blessing of management for my decision, I was still curious to see how the members of this core unit, the men and women who were there every night doing their various production jobs, would take it. I scanned the faces around the table to see understanding nods and heard a few, "Well, we'll miss ya in San Antonio." It was gratifying. A number of them came up afterward to say they understood the situation and were cool with my decision. Then a member of our public relations staff took me aside and said that while he understood, others in the media might not.

"Will you be available to talk to TV writers if you skip game seven? They'll want to know why you're not there for a game that big."

My response was immediate.

"You can give them my number, and I'll tell them that I never want my son to think he came in second to a basketball game."

In my Dallas hotel room about five hours before game time, I had a lot of things bouncing around in my brain. I was putting the finishing touches on my notes for the show and reassuring myself that missing game seven, if there was one, was the right thing to do. Of course, that bump near my left ear was still there, and I had thought about it every day for four months now. I needed to call home and talk to Cheryl. She couldn't help with my pregame prep, and I still hadn't told her about the bump, but she could certainly reassure me about game seven versus Eric's graduation.

We had talked about it at the outset and never really revisited it, because I had made my decision. But there was one phrase I wanted to hear from her before our phone call was over. I was not going to request it or coax her into saying it, but man, did I want to hear it. I told her about the morning production meeting and about PR telling me I might have to defend myself with writers. As we wrapped up the call, I said, "Well, no matter what happens tonight, I'll see you tomorrow."

And then she said it. "Hey . . . you're a good dad."

You see, in the course of being a parent, there have been times I've felt overmatched or simply not qualified for the job.

You think you're doing the right thing when you're trying to handle a problem, and you completely botch it and make it worse. You don't say the right words in a given situation, or you remain silent when you should speak up, and instead of putting out a fire, you pour gasoline on it. Cheryl's always had a knack for knowing exactly when to reassure me that I'm not a lost cause. And when she says, "You're a good dad," it is good for my soul.

American Airlines Center was rockin' late in the third quarter of game six. The Mavs had a fifteen-point lead and were one quarter and change from forcing game seven in San Antonio with a trip to the NBA Finals on the line. Honestly, at that point, I knew I'd be missing it for Eric's graduation, and I was good with that. Cheryl's words that afternoon had given me peace.

Then Steve Kerr happened.

Steve played in more than nine hundred NBA games but started only thirty times. He was a valuable drop-dead shooter off the bench in his eleven seasons in the league. He had four championship rings, three of them from his time on the Michael Jordan–led Bulls team, though it was Kerr himself who had hit the championship-winning jumper for Chicago in 1997. It was my good fortune to later work with him, as he joined Turner Sports after his retirement. He is simply a down-to-earth, genuine, good guy . . . who can really shoot. He was looking for ring number five and his second with the Spurs in 2003, and the clock on his career was winding down.

He had seen three minutes of action through five games of this Western Conference Final. But late in the third quarter,

Spurs coach Gregg Popovich, looking for some kind of spark with his team down by double digits, summoned Kerr. He took his first shot of the series, a three-pointer with 1:40 to go in the third, and it went down, cutting Dallas's lead to nine. But it was back to thirteen going into the fourth quarter. The Spurs cut Dallas's lead to single digits in no time, and when Stephen Jackson hit back-to-back threes, we had a game. And then, like I said, Steve Kerr happened. A three-pointer to tie the game at seventy-one, another for the lead, and yet another for an eight-point advantage with five minutes left. San Antonio would win by twelve. Steve Kerr played thirteen minutes, scored twelve points, and didn't miss a shot.

They held the Western Conference Championship trophy presentation in a meeting room near the locker rooms in Dallas because the road team had won, and there weren't many fans in Dallas interested in watching the Spurs celebrate. During the commercial break before the ceremony, as I got ready to interview Steve Kerr, I said, "Hey, Ted!" Steve laughed. When we had spoken earlier in the week about his lack of minutes in the series, he had said some of his teammates had been referring to him as Ted Williams. The news had carried stories about the baseball legend being frozen after his passing, and now a few of Kerr's buddies had joked that they'd have to break the ice around Steve if he got a chance to play.

Somebody took a picture of us during the interview, and it was later mailed to me, and I still have it. When I look at it, I remember that night . . . one of those incredible unscripted play-off games that turned on the performance of a guy who was ready when his name was called. And I'm reminded of a moment in which I got the best of both worlds. I wouldn't have to miss a second of work, and I would get to proudly watch my first child, Eric, walk onstage, turn his tassel, and begin the next chapter of his life. And I remember a phone call and a wife's encouragement. A blackberry.

At this point, you may be thinking, and rightfully so, that with our NBA coverage finished and a little vacation time coming, it was time for me to see a doctor about whatever was lurking just below the surface near my left ear. I always had an excuse for putting it off. Fear and denial were winning out over common sense. We had a family week at the beach coming up in June before I would leave for England and Turner's first venture into the Open Championship in July, followed by the PGA Championship at Oak Hill in Rochester, New York, in August. So I made a little deal with myself and vowed that if that "thing" hadn't gone away by the time the PGA Championship was over, I would go to the doctor. But for now, it was time to pack for England.

Ever seen photos of the white cliffs of Dover? Spectacular. With their chalky composition, they stand out brilliantly on the English shoreline, and to many people there, they stand as a monument to freedom, not unlike the way the Statue of Liberty is revered by Americans. Long ago they stood as a fortress for English troops protecting the homeland against invaders, and they were celebrated in the song "The White Cliffs of Dover" during World War II.

My hotel room for the Open Championship was fourteen miles from the golf course. It was tiny. It had no air-conditioning. On the sun-drenched, cloudless day I arrived, I opened the window in the room, hoping a stray breeze might somehow make the room a little less like a sauna. And when I opened that window, I saw, not half a mile away, the white cliffs of Dover. Spectacular indeed.

In the three days leading up to the Open, I made time each day, when I wasn't at Royal St. George's preparing for our broadcast, to go running near the cliffs, which were even more breathtaking when viewed from close range. I love runs like that. When I'm not trying to push through fatigue or wondering which hurts more, my left ankle or my right calf, I use that time to sort of soak in God's creation. I do a lot of thinking, a lot of praying—for my family thousands of miles away, for friends who might be facing tough situations. And as I ran down well-worn paths, and on the grassy plateau above the cliffs, and past the South Foreland Lighthouse, I'll be honest, I was praying that everything was all right with my health.

Sure, I'll remember that week for the stunning performance of Ben Curtis, who rose from anonymity to claim the famed Claret Jug, which goes to the winner. And I'll remember Tiger Woods teeing off in round one and promptly losing his ball in the ankle-high rough to the right of the first fairway. And I'll remember thinking our TV tower was going to blow over in frighteningly high winds. But in some odd way, and I guess it's because I'm wired a little differently, the first things that come to mind when I think about our first Open Championship are the white cliffs of Dover and the song of hope they once inspired. Because at that time in my life, I was five months deep into a period marked by anxiety, fear, and still . . . hope.

9

Tough Conversations

REMEMBER THAT DEAL I had made with myself—the one about seeing the doctor if that "thing" still wasn't gone by the time the PGA Championship was over? It was time. The PGA had ended dramatically on Sunday, August 17, with one of the greatest seven irons struck by a player . . . ever. Shaun Micheel had come to the seventy-second hole nursing a one-shot lead over Chad Campbell and had watched his tee shot bounce in the fairway and into the first cut of rough 174 yards from the pin. And that's when he launched that seven iron. With the ball in flight, Micheel's caddy could be heard saying those two words the pros love to say when a shot has a chance to be not just close but *really* close.

"Be right!"

Jim Nantz of CBS picked it up from there. "Is it right? It could be in!" And as the ball came to rest just inches from the cup, he said, "Add that to PGA Championship lore!" It was the perfect call of the perfect golf shot. Micheel tapped

119

the ball in to seal the deal and would have his name engraved on the Wanamaker Trophy with all the other winners of the PGA Championship. This was the drama of sports at its highest level. Meanwhile, my own personal drama was about to unfold, quickly, over the next four days.

One of my neighbors in Braselton, Georgia, is an orthopedist. Dr. Rhett Rainey is a guy we can call if one of the kids breaks a bone or sprains something or if Cheryl or I suffer some kind of "weekend warrior" injury that reminds us we're not as young as we think we are. On that Monday evening, Dr. Rainey was in his front yard, and I said, "Rhett, I need your advice. I've got this thing near my left ear," and I demonstrated for him how it appeared when I moved my mouth to the right, as I'd done so many times while shaving. "Whaddaya think, Doc, is this just a normal thing that'll go away in time, something you see a lot?" Obviously, my line of questioning was all geared toward a best-case scenario. Must have been a rather unique snapshot for anybody who happened to be driving or walking past at that moment—me with my mouth extending toward my right shoulder and him running his hand from my left ear down my cheekbone.

"Yeah, you need to have this looked at."

"What do you think? Any ideas?"

"Not really something I deal with on a regular basis. I've got a good friend who's an ear, nose, and throat specialist, and I could connect you guys, but you need to get this taken care of."

I finally told Cheryl what I had kept to myself for the past several months, told her about my conversation with Rhett, and explained that the only reason I had kept it to myself was to keep her from worrying about it. I got a scolding. I don't remember the conversation exactly, but it went something like this.

"Why did you wait so long to tell me? I'm your wife. I've been your wife for twenty years, and we don't hide anything."

"But I was just—"

"I'm your wife. If there's a problem or something that might be a problem, we talk about it."

"But it may have been nothing to—"

"I'm your wife. I love you. If there's something wrong, I want to know about it. I want to help you deal with it. We go through everything together."

I was in the doctor's office (Rhett's ENT friend) the next afternoon.

A benign parotid tumor. That's what the doctor told me after feeling around on the left side of my face and asking a series of questions about how long it had been since I had first noticed the bump and whether there was any pain associated with it, which there was not. And of course, my question was, "What the heck is a benign parotid tumor?" He explained it was a tumor in the salivary glands. I didn't like the sound of the word *tumor*, but I did like the sound of the word *benign*, and I loved the fact that the word *cancer* had not been spoken. So my next question was, "How do we get rid of it?" He explained that if it were to increase in size to the point that it had to be surgically removed, it would be a fairly commonplace procedure but would involve working close to the facial nerve, which calls for a very precise surgical technique. If the surgeon should nick the facial nerve, he told me, I would lose muscular control on that side of my face. That would mean everything from speech to smiling to closing my left eye would be affected, possibly permanently.

It was a frightening proposition, especially for a guy who makes his living on television, and while he assured me that those instances are rare, I was spooked by that worst-case scenario. Then he said that while it was his opinion I had a benign parotid tumor, he would be happy to set me up with another doctor to get a second opinion. I agreed and went home to wait for a phone call to tell me where and when this next appointment would happen. That word came on Wednesday, August 20. I had an appointment at the Emory University Hospital with Dr. William Grist. What caught me off guard was that his office was right next to the Winship Cancer Institute.

Thursday, August 21, 2003. Our twenty-first wedding anniversary. While Cheryl went to work, I sat in Dr. Grist's office and heard many of the same questions I had been asked just two days before, but then there came a new one.

"Have you had a fine-needle biopsy?"

"A what?"

"On Tuesday, did the doctor draw a sample from the area of the tumor?"

"No, he seemed pretty convinced this was a benign parotid tumor, and we discussed the possibility of surgery at some point and the complications that might arise."

"Well, before we go any further, I think we need a fine-needle biopsy."

So I made my way from his office to building B of the Emory clinic, where Dr. Melinda Lewis, a pathologist, greeted me with a smile and a friendly, "This won't really hurt much," and in went the needle about a half inch from my left ear. She was right—it didn't hurt, and in a matter of seconds, she walked into an adjoining room with the sample she had collected. A few minutes passed, and she returned with another needle.

"Sorry, I'd just like to do this one more time if that's okay."

"No problem."

Except there was a problem.

When she returned from the adjoining room after studying the second sample, she explained that what she saw concerned her. Both samples were filled with lymphocytes, a type of white blood cell that grows and multiplies uncontrollably. She had seen this countless times in her twenty years at Emory, and in the most compassionate way possible, but without sugarcoating it, she told me that while the samples would need to be further analyzed, it appeared to her trained eye that I had non-Hodgkin's lymphoma. Cancer. Me. Cancer. That word hung in the air as we sat in absolute silence for what seemed an eternity but was probably no more than ten seconds. And then we just sat and talked for the next twenty minutes.

Dr. Lewis got her bachelor's degree at the University of Michigan and went to med school at Emory, graduating from both magna cum laude, and I am certain that somewhere along that path she aced a course in doctor-patient relations, if there is such a thing. Or maybe she's just Mother Teresa with a stethoscope. That twenty-minute conversation, during which we talked about everything from coming to grips with the diagnosis, to sharing the news with my family, to what kind of treatment I might expect to go through, to maintaining a positive attitude, was the best medicine I could have gotten at the time. She walked me to the door that led to the parking lot, and rather than shaking her hand, I gave her a hug and said thanks. She looked me square in the eye and with a smile said simply, "Hey, it's gonna be okay." And somehow I knew it would.

I was dozing on the couch that night when Cheryl came home from a workday that included an event that evening. I knew her first question would be about my visit to Emory, and I was dreading having to answer it. While Dr. Lewis had so expertly laid it all out in front of me that afternoon, I was holding tightly to the slim chance that the rest of the testing on the samples she had taken would reveal there had been a mistake. She told me Dr. Grist would be calling on Friday with the results.

"Hey, hon. So how did it go today? What did they say?"

"Well, they stuck a needle into the tumor and drew out a sample. They need to run it through a few machines, and they'll call with the results tomorrow. Hey, you look tired. We could both use a good night's sleep."

I know, I know. Cheryl had already been hurt by my five months of keeping that undiagnosed "thing" to myself, and here I was again—telling part of the story. I'm sorry—I just couldn't bring myself to say "cancer" at that very moment. I knew at some point the next day I would get a call from Dr. Grist, and it would more than likely support what Dr. Lewis had found, but what if it didn't? Then what? I would have rocked Cheryl's world with that one word—*cancer*—only to find out the next day that somehow, amazingly, it wasn't. I was rationalizing my silence to the point of exhaustion. Today, nearly fifteen years later, I'm still ashamed of that. Cheryl deserved better.

The phone call came around 6:30 Friday evening as we sat eating dinner—Cheryl and me and Carmen and Michael and Eric, who had come home from college for the weekend.

I excused myself from the table and hurried into another room, answering on the third ring.

"Ernie, this is Dr. Grist. The results of your fine-needle biopsy are in. I know you spoke with Dr. Lewis yesterday, and what she told you then is true. This is non-Hodgkin's lymphoma. It's a form of blood cancer, but I want to point out that it is a very treatable form of cancer, and I'm putting you in the care of one of the best oncologists anywhere. His name is Dr. Leonard Heffner."

"So what do I do now?"

"I'm in the process of setting up another appointment next week. We'll have to run some tests and have you scanned so we can determine if the cancer has spread to other parts of your body. Only then will we know what course of action to take in terms of treatment."

As I hung up the phone and headed back toward the kitchen, Eric and Carmen met me in the hallway on their way out the door.

"Hey, Dad, we're goin' to Blockbuster to get a movie. Any requests?"

"Something funny."

Cheryl knew who the phone call was from. She waited for the door to close behind Eric and Carmen before she spoke. "Well?"

"That was Dr. Grist from Emory."

"I figured. And . . ."

"And, Cheryl, it's worse than we thought. It's cancer. Non-Hodgkin's lymphoma."

I wish that moment on no man. Its pain is indescribable. Telling my wife of twenty-one years was a thousand times worse than hearing the word from Dr. Lewis the day before.

We stood in the middle of the den holding each other and sobbing. By the time Carmen and Eric returned from the video store, we had fought to regain our composure. The rest of the night was a blur. We watched the movie the kids had picked out, but for the life of me I can't remember what it was. All I remember was lying next to Cheryl later that night, both of us staring at the ceiling and wondering aloud how this was all going to play out, how we were going to tell the kids the next day, how we were going to tell our parents, and how lucky we were to have each other for this unscripted chapter of our lives.

There were several difficult conversations to come. How do you tell your kids that Dad has cancer? How do you tell your mom and dad? There is no "easy start" guide like you find with a new piece of electronics. Simply charge this piece . . . plug this in . . . create a password . . . connect to Wi-Fi . . . boom! You're up and runnin'. Nothing prepares you for the look on your kids' faces when you say, "I need you guys to have a seat. There's something we need to talk about as a family." They know this isn't going to be about a vacation we want to take when school's out. This isn't going to be about how they've been neglecting their jobs around the house or how they may have mistreated their brothers or sisters in a weak moment. So what was this going to be about? I could tell by the expressionless faces of Eric (eighteen), Maggie (sixteen), Michael (fifteen), and Carmen (nine) staring at me that they knew this was different. This was serious. And so all I could do was shoot straight.

"Gang, this isn't easy for me. Eric and Carmen, you know I took a phone call at dinner last night. Well, it was from a doctor at Emory. There's been a bump on the left side of my face near my ear for the last six months, and I finally had it checked out this week. The doctor was calling to tell me that it's cancer. It's something they call non-Hodgkin's lymphoma."

Immediately, they were in tears. At least Eric, Maggie, and Carmen were. I've already told you about Michael's history. The gravity of the situation never really registered with him, probably because this family meeting had nothing to do with cars. When the hugs were done and the kids were finished wiping their eyes with Kleenex or shirtsleeves, I continued.

"Look, that's basically all I know right now. The doctor says it's a very treatable form of cancer. In fact, for what it's worth, he said, 'If you have to have cancer, it's the best kind to have.' I'll have to go back to Emory next week for some more tests, and then we'll know what I have to do. But this isn't about me. This is about us. This is about all of us pulling together to get through this. If you're worried about me, talk to me about it, not somebody from school who might have a story that scares you. We will get through this."

Then we held hands and said a prayer, asking God for courage and strength and comfort and healing. And then we hugged some more.

My mother, Lois, is a cancer survivor. Breast cancer, colon cancer—she beat them both. She also knows the reality of hearing that one of her kids has cancer. My oldest sister, Dawn, was diagnosed with breast cancer in her twenties. She, too, is a survivor. Now two days after that gut-wrenching session with my kids, I was driving to my parents' house to deliver my news. She reacted as any mom would, but it was with shock and sadness tinged with the resolve of somebody who had been down that road and made it. I told her that she and my sister had set the bar pretty high, and I was determined to join them in the ranks of cancer survivors.

My father wasn't home at the time. He was playing in a charity golf tournament that day, ironically, at a course just two miles from my house. He and his foursome were putting on the fourteenth green in one of those scramble formats where the quality of the golf pales in comparison to the sheer fun of the day. My dad was the "celebrity" in the group—a baseball player and broadcaster who would enthrall his group with stories of his playing days and all those nights in the broadcast booth. Dad must have played in a thousand of those tournaments, raising money for various charities, and to this day men come up to me out of the blue and tell me of a time when they were lucky enough to be in a foursome with the old right-hander—and how they will never forget his stories, his friendliness, and how he treated each of them as if they were lifelong buddies. That never surprised me. It was one of those life lessons Dad had instilled in me without even trying to teach me. I just watched him. And hearing from men who had been impacted by his genuine kindness simply cemented the importance of character. All I ever wanted to do was be the best imitation of my father I could possibly be. That's tough duty.

And so was this. I approached my father as he and the others made their way to their carts to head to the next tee.

"How you hittin' 'em, Big Guy?"

"Oh, I don't know . . . fellas, what are we . . . five, six under? We might be in the running for a bag of tees at the awards barbecue."

"Think you might have a few minutes to stop by the house when you're finished?"

"Sure . . . what's up?"

"Aw, nothin' really . . . just got something to talk about if you can stop by for a few minutes."

"Just got a few holes left, and then I'm gonna emcee the awards thing, and then I'll swing by."

I can't really remember ever seeing my dad, the old, proud marine, cry. As much as I'd always tried to emulate his character, we couldn't be more dissimilar in that department. When Harry Bailey comes home to help his brother in the classic *It's a Wonderful Life* and says, "Here's to my big brother, George, the richest man in town," I get that lump in my throat and my eyes get all glassy. When the father and son play catch in the final scene of *Field of Dreams* or when Steve Martin sees his daughter's life pass before his eyes in *Father of the Bride*, I'm a teary-eyed, sniffling wreck. My dad stayed true to form late that afternoon when I told him I had cancer. And for once, in the midst of the most emotional of moments for me, I broke form. Didn't shed a tear. We locked eyes, told each other how much we loved each other. I vowed to follow the lead of my mother and sister and kick the crap out of this disease that had suddenly invaded our lives again.

Now there was one more conversation I needed to have.

10

Trust God . . . Period

BEFORE I WENT BACK to Emory that week in 2003, I needed to sit down with Kevin Myers. Kevin is my pastor, and six years earlier he had led me down a life-altering path.

He introduced me to Jesus Christ.

At that time, in the fall of 1997, Cheryl and I were busy raising four kids, and I was busy trying to make a name for myself as a sportscaster on the national level. In all honesty, the latter is what was driving my very existence. My identity was tied more to that career quest than my status as a husband and father. I was raised Catholic and was your run-of-the-mill churchgoing altar boy as a kid. A kid who quickly drifted away from anything church related or God related when I went off to college at the University of Georgia. Sunday mornings were designed to sleep in and shake off the effects of too much Saturday night fun, not to set an alarm clock so I could hit the 9:00 mass. On occasion I'd go to church with my folks on a weekend at home, but it had been so long that I hardly remembered when to stand, sit, or kneel.

So knowing that background, we fast-forward twenty years or so. It's 1997, and Cheryl and I have this great family, a beautiful home, and good jobs, and in our minds, God has had nothing to do with it. We had tried a couple churches along the way, but nothing long term, and had gone back to our norm of leisurely Sunday mornings. But many of our kids' friends were going to church every Sunday, and they were asking Eric and Maggie, in particular, since they were the older of our children, why they didn't go to church. Eric and Maggie in turn asked us, and we really didn't have an answer. So Cheryl and I had this fairly deep discussion and decided it might be good if the kids had some consistent exposure to this whole "spiritual thing" and we would scout out a few potential landing spots.

One of those was a church called Crossroads. It was a nondenominational, Bible-based church we had driven past a million times, sometimes wondering aloud, "What is that place with the blue roof?" It didn't really look like a church. There was an office trailer at one end of the parking lot, a playground at the other, and in between was a stone building with a blue roof.

On one Sunday afternoon, the parking lot virtually empty, I stopped by to see if a door was open, hoping maybe I could grab some printed information and take it home. Turns out there was a church member there that day, and he explained that Crossroads was just about ten years old. When it started, they had held services at a movie theater for the twenty-five or so people who attended and later in a jazzercise studio. Now they had this real building for the 150 or so who called it their church home. I had no idea when I stood there chatting with this stranger that over the next twenty years this Crossroads would change locations again and again to bigger, more accommodating spaces, would change its name to 12 Stone, and would serve upward of twenty-five thousand people every weekend at a main campus with half a dozen satellite locations. All I knew right then was that this little place with the blue roof had a service for adults and a separate one for the kids at the same time in one of the meeting rooms there. This sounded like it might be worth a try. And remember, Cheryl and I were doing this for the kids. Right.

The first service we attended was unlike anything either of us had ever experienced, and we weren't sure that was a good thing. There was no organ music. There was a band. There were no time-honored hymns being sung. There was something I later learned was called contemporary Christian music being sung, and people were clapping along with it. Let's just say my comfort level was not exactly high at this point. There were no suits and ties. There were jeans. And there was no priest. There was this guy, Kevin Myers. He was the most gifted communicator and teacher I had ever heard, and it appeared he knew the Bible back and forth. I hadn't opened one in about a quarter of a century, but that day I was immersed in it, because if you didn't own a Bible, you were welcome to take the one where you were sitting. I remember taking notes on the handout we were given at the door as if this information was going to be on some final exam I had to prepare for. Which I guess is kind of true.

Anyway, Kevin posed a couple questions that day. "Who's the provider in your family?" and "What are you pursuing, happiness or wholeness?" Well, I had this. (1) I'm the provider, and (2) happiness. Seems I was 0 for 2. Over the next few weeks, we explored these questions at Crossroads, and long story short, a light just seemed to go on for me. And it was shining on a life that was in need of recalibration. I was living such a me-centered existence that naturally I viewed myself as the provider, and I was all about the next thing that would make me happy—something I would buy, some recognition of my work that would let me throw back my head and puff out my chest and say, "Look at me!" And now here I was on what used to be laid-back Sunday mornings at home taking notes about God the provider and this Jesus, who came to serve, not to be served, and how happiness is okay, but wholeness is what it's all about, and the only way to be the husband and father I need to be is to have a heavenly Father who's directing my steps, and the only way to do that is to surrender to the God who made me, who sent his Son to die for my sins so that I can be forgiven and have a relationship with God through Jesus. Shoot, I even started clapping along with those songs that were now becoming familiar. After about a month, I cornered Kevin after a service.

"Hey, do you wanna grab lunch one of these days? I don't know how to put this exactly, but God's messin' with me."

"I'd love to. How about Wednesday?"

Wednesday, December 10, 1997, became my "spiritual birthday," the day Kevin and I sat at an O'Charley's restaurant in Lawrenceville, Georgia, talking about where I had been in my life, where I saw myself going, and this kind of gnawing feeling that there had to be more to my existence than my job and its stranglehold on me. He said four words I still remember. "You're a prayer away." So that's what we did. Right there at the table. Prayed to turn a me-centered life into a Christ-centered life. Took about twenty seconds to say a prayer that changed me for eternity. Blackberry.

Now I just had to live it out.

Here's a story you may find amusing. At least it is now. It was sort of gut-wrenching at the time. The 1998 PGA Championship was going to be played in Seattle at Sahalee Country Club, and so several weeks before, media day was held. It gives the national golf press and the TV crews from Turner and CBS a chance to play the course and talk to the course superintendent and others as part of our preparation for the championship. I had been a new Christian for about six months and had, I guess you could say, a peaceful, *uneasy* feeling in some ways when it came to going public with my faith.

There were days when I'd be walking into a Family Christian Store to buy some music or a book and would actually break into a sweat thinking somebody was going to recognize me and ask me what I was doing there or, heaven forbid, quiz me on something biblical. One day I bought one of those Christian fish symbols to put on my bumper and then stood in the parking lot for ten minutes getting up the nerve to stick it on. I was worried about what co-workers might think and say, like, "What's Ernie doing driving around with *that* on his bumper? Shoot, I once heard the guy drop four F-bombs when we ran the wrong highlight in postgame."

So back to Sahalee. I was standing in my hotel room that morning getting ready to head to the golf course with my buddies from Turner, and I decided this was the day I would wear for the first time in my life a WWJD (What would Jesus do?) bracelet. The fish on my bumper hadn't raised any questions, so now I would take the next step. I took the elevator to the lobby, saw my co-workers waiting with their golf clubs, and promptly took the elevator back up to my room and took off the bracelet. Then I put it back on. I took the elevator back downstairs and joined up with my buddies, and off we went to play eighteen. I will admit that during the course of the day, anytime I'd be talking to somebody I would be watching their eyes to see if they were noticing what was on my wrist. During those hours on the golf course, it hit me. Here I was, having made a decision to put an end to a me-centered life, and all I had been doing all day was thinking about . . . me. You could have hit me right between the eyes with a four iron and it wouldn't have had the impact of that simple realization.

This life was not going to be about what I wore or what I put on my bumper. It was going to be about the way I lived each and every day. And the only way to live a life of faith was to be in tune with the Holy Spirit. It was about being obedient to a voice that wasn't mine.

I had help in this journey from men just like me—fathers, husbands, businessmen. Fifteen or twenty of us would gather at Crossroads at 6:00 a.m. every Friday for Bible study. Men like Corey Baker and Doug Moran would share their stories, we would dive into the Word, and I would gain a whole new appreciation for the Bible. It wasn't this antiquated bunch of stories that had no relevance in modern times, as had been my opinion for ages. It was a book *for the ages*, a love letter from God to his people packed with practical, everyday wisdom. I can never thank guys like Corey and Doug enough for the hours they spent pouring what they had learned through the years into me. And the same can be said of the members of the study I joined a couple years later and am still attending on Thursday mornings going on fifteen years now.

Tim Cash started the group. He was a pitcher whose arm problems kept him from reaching the major leagues as a player. But he reached the majors as a leader of Baseball Chapel, holding Sunday services before games and mentoring countless players, leading many to a new life in Christ. He invited me to join his group, which met in the back of a barbecue restaurant outside Atlanta. Among our number are a couple guys whose names you'll recognize right off the bat: Jeff Foxworthy, the comedian and TV host, and Hall of Fame pitcher John Smoltz. There are other former professional baseball and football players in the group, along with a few local businessmen. But when we walk into that room, nobody has a professional title.

We're there to grow as men of God. It's that simple. Sure, while we're devouring bacon and eggs and grits and biscuits and gravy, we'll hear Smoltzy tell a story or two about games he'll never forget, and Jeff will trot out some new material and a "you might be a redneck" joke or two. But when breakfast is done, we get down to business. And that means helping a brother through a tough time, or holding each other accountable to stay on the right path, or breaking down biblical teaching we can't quite get a handle on. (That happens a lot with our crew.) So to Tim and Jeff and John, and Chuck Scott, Todd Peterson, Lowry Robinson, Tom Tabor, Lester Archambeau, John Burrough, Mark Parker, Paul Byrd, Todd Greene, Bruce Coker, Brett Butler, Todd Weiner, Mike McCoy, Trey Miller, and the others who will give me an incredibly hard time for leaving them off this list—thanks, fellas. My life would not be the same without you.

Oh, and in case you're wondering, Cheryl turned her life over too, though it took substantially longer than it did for me. Cheryl's a deep thinker. (I stay more in the shallow end.) She accepts very little at face value, and when it came to this matter of faith, she wanted proof. I made a decision for Christ knowing I still had a ton to learn, while my wife wanted to learn as much as she could before making any kind of commitment.

There were passages in the Bible she could not agree with, and there were stories she could not believe. Kevin made regular visits to our house after December 10 to walk us through the Bible, from Genesis to Revelation, and in the course of those kitchen table discussions, there were moments of clear realization and outright skepticism.

Let me be totally honest here. It got messy around our house. While Cheryl could appreciate the step I had taken, she wasn't there yet. I'm trying to clean up my language, trying to set aside time to get into the Bible, stopping by a Family Christian Store to buy Steven Curtis Chapman CDs and a fish for the back of my car, and she's looking at me and asking, "Are you the same guy I married fifteen years ago?" It's hard when you're coming at something as pivotal as faith from different angles. Kevin was in the middle of this, providing not only biblical perspective but also commonsense talk about life—our lives.

"Look at where you've been—these adoptions, the way you care for this special-needs child," Kevin would say. "I'm telling you, your lives reflect the love of Jesus Christ more than the lives of so many people who have identified as Christians their entire lives. Let's not get hung up on labels. Let's just get intentional about your faith. I'm telling you, you're living

Christian lives, but you just don't know it. And even though you weren't paying any attention to God, he was paying attention to you. How'd you wind up at that particular orphanage in Romania, Cheryl? Ernie, why'd you immediately say, 'Bring him home' when your wife described this kid's condition? Did those things just randomly happen, or was this the work of a Creator who orchestrates life in ways we can't begin to understand? That's how the Holy Spirit works, guys—gives you just a nudge, Cheryl, and says, 'That's the boy . . . the one with the blond hair . . . the one who can't walk or talk . . . that's the one.' That's the Holy Spirit who whispers in your ear, Ernie, 'Bring him home' at the very moment your wife is asking for an answer over a static-filled phone line from Romania. Now if your answer to those questions is that it just somehow happened, we need to go back to square one. But if you believe there's a grand design being played out before our very eyes, then let's press on."

And we did. And we hit brick walls. And we obliterated some. And we agreed to disagree on some things, but on others there was firm common ground that steadied us, like the belief that this life isn't all there is. That there is something more. That there is life everlasting. That this family we have on earth, which includes a Romanian orphan with a fatal disease, will someday be reunited in heaven. It was that eternal perspective that for Cheryl trumped all those things she was struggling to wrap her head around. Her spiritual birthday was March 25, 1998.

Blackberry . . . the size of Montana.

So now you know why Kevin Myers was the other person I needed to speak with. He had been a spiritual mentor to me for going on six years now. He made himself available for the multitude of questions I would throw at him and always had a scriptural basis to underscore his response. I valued his friendship. We were both husbands and fathers. We were roughly the same age. I was a little older—he was a good bit wiser. He had a much better handle on the stuff that really matters, and I was trying to get there.

So now we were sitting in a local Starbucks talking about how having a doctor speak one particular *c* word can pretty much knock your world off its axis, and was it okay that I wanted to punch God right in the nose? We began to unpack what I said I believed, going all the way back to that day in December 1997. Was this diagnosis going to shake my faith to its core, or was my faith going to carry me through this trial? Did I truly believe what the apostle Paul wrote in his letter to the Romans, that in *all* things God works for the good of those who believe? He didn't say all things *except* non-Hodgkin's lymphoma. Yeah, I believed that. We talked about Job in the Old Testament having his life turned upside down, yet through it all, though he openly questioned what God was doing or was allowing to happen, he never lost his faith.

"In times like this, you have a couple options," Kevin told me. "You can turn *on* God, or you can turn *to* God."

We talked about the ninth chapter in the Gospel of John where the disciples asked about the blind man by the side of the road. Why had this happened to him? Who had sinned, this man or his parents? Jesus's response was, in essence, "You're asking the wrong question. It's not *why* this happened but *how* God is going to use it for his glory." I got that. But the moment of that heart-to-heart talk in the middle of a busy coffee shop that would mark my life was yet to come.

Kevin pulled a pen from his pocket, grabbed a light brown Starbucks napkin, and wrote down one word.

"EJ, this whole thing is about this: trust." He held up the napkin to show me and then went back to writing.

"Is it going to be trust with a question mark? Is it going to be 'I'll trust God *if* the next test at Emory comes back the way I want it to'? Or is it going to be trust. Period. You trusted him with your life six years ago. It's easy to trust him when things are going great and you're being blessed with good things left and right. How does that trust feel right now, while you're looking up from this valley you've never been in?"

And that's why I had to talk to Kevin Myers. And that's why to this day, whenever I send an email, my signature at the bottom of the message looks like this:

Ernie Johnson Jr.
Trust God . . . Period.

11

You May Have Cancer, but It Doesn't Have You

"YOU LOOK WAY TOO GOOD to be hangin' out in here."

That's what the lab technician told me prior to one of the early scans I had to determine the extent of the cancer that had invaded my body. Cheryl and I felt the same way. The whole thing was surreal from the moment we walked into Emory's Winship Cancer Institute. My wife and I just stared at each other as we sat in the office of the financial consultant who was talking to us about insurance coverage and the like. We couldn't believe we were sitting there and having this conversation. We couldn't believe I was now part of the population we were seeing in the waiting room. There were people wearing surgical masks. Some were bald. Some looked too weak to stand, while others were pacing. And over this entire scene hung a distinct feeling of anxiety.

One of these days would I also be wearing "that look" of those for whom the cancer battle had taken a visible toll?

At this point, I looked a lot more like the friends and family of patients who were getting checkups or preparing for another round of chemotherapy. The difference was that I was wearing the Emory patient bracelet and was about to undergo a series of tests to determine the extent of my non-Hodgkin's lymphoma.

"Remember, you may have cancer, but it doesn't have you."

Again, words of that lab tech reminding me that my attitude in the course of this unscripted journey was going to be vital. Years later it is advice I've shared with countless cancer patients who face the same uncertainty and apprehension I felt. For me, it meant I was going to fight with every ounce of strength I had. I was going to "trust God . . . period," and I was going to remain positive. That's not the easiest thing in the world to do. Not when a nurse is sticking an enormous needle into your hip bone as she extracts a bone marrow sample. That was just one of the tests I underwent on that first day. There were others, such as the CT scan that helped doctors determine the stage at which the cancer had been diagnosed, but that particular bone marrow biopsy stood out above the rest.

Lying facedown on a table, I could hear the sounds of the nurse preparing the needle and syringe. I could feel the area near my lower back being prepped. I heard her explanation of what was about to happen, that I would feel "tremendous pressure." She wasn't kidding. The pain and the pressure on my lower back were intense. And then there was the sound. I don't know how best to describe it, but it sounded to me like one of those bicycle tire pumps being pushed down and then pulled back up again—the needle going in and the bone marrow sample being withdrawn time and again. I was gripping the sides of the table for all I was worth, and while I felt like yelling, all I can recall is grunting, not unlike the sound you might make while lifting weights. I tried to block out the pain by silently reciting the lyrics of a song written by Bebo Norman called "I Am" (an Old Testament reference to God's name Yahweh, meaning "I am"). The song's message is that no matter what you might be going through, in your household, in your job, in your marriage, or in my case, in your doctor's office going through a procedure you think will never end, you're not alone. "I am in the marrow and the blood" is the line that resonated with me, because that's right where I was that afternoon on that table with that God.

It was over in a matter of ten to fifteen minutes, and then the waiting game began. The results of that day of testing would be analyzed, and a few days later we would have an assessment. My oncologist, Dr. Leonard Heffner, notified me that I had stage 2 (out of 4) follicular non-Hodgkin's lymphoma. It was, he pointed out, not an aggressive form of cancer, that it was present in my lymph nodes but not in my bone marrow, and that while it was not *curable*, it was very *treatable*, and our goal would be to get it into remission. He pointed out that many patients with this type of cancer live long lives. And we talked about treatment. There would be none at this point because aside from the swelling near my left ear and a few other spots, I was basically asymptomatic—meaning I wasn't feeling sick. In his opinion, we should take the approach of "watchful waiting." I would go to Winship three times a year, and at each visit, my blood would be tested and Dr. Heffner would feel up and down my neck, under my armpits, and around my groin, all areas where there are lymph nodes, to see if anything had changed in size from the previous visit. We followed this regimen for nearly three years.

In 2006, things changed. The swelling near my left ear and on the right side of my neck had grown more pronounced, and I had grown more self-conscious about how I looked on the air. I would stand in front of the mirror before I went on and look at my face from different angles. I would wonder what the makeup artist was thinking but not saying. I would wonder if the camera operators shooting me during the show were noticing that something was different. The tipping point came at the NBA All-Star Game in February 2006 in Houston.

I was honored that the league asked me to welcome the crowd to the game from center court and then introduce the starting lineups. In a phone call with Cheryl, I asked her to record it so I could watch it the next night when I was home. We watched the recording together and both saw the same thing. It was time for me to go public with the news I had cancer. Dr. Heffner and I met and considered my options. If I wanted to begin chemotherapy at this point, I could, but it was not imperative. I still felt great and told him I preferred to wait until we were finished with our NBA coverage in May. The message I wanted to send to viewers was that while I had received a cancer diagnosis, it didn't mean I needed to go into hiding. I wanted to keep working and then start treatment.

By this time, two and a half years since I had been diagnosed, only a few people knew what I was going through—my family, a couple close friends, and a few executives at work. But now everyone was going to know. An hour before we hit the air for our first show after the All-Star break, I called Charles Barkley and Kenny Smith into my office separately to let them know what I was dealing with. My news was met with stunned silence and shaking heads. Both said, "If you need anything, or if your family needs anything, just ask."

My only request of both was that we not let my news affect the show's dynamic. We had made a living the past six years doing a lighthearted basketball show—no place to be if you're thin-skinned, since we were constantly jabbing each other, tossing insults at each other, and generally having a full-court free-for-all. To each I said, "Look, this can't change the way we do our show. I don't want you to lay off me because I have cancer. Things have to continue the way they always have. It's one of the reasons people love the show."

That night on our pregame show, we spent the first segment talking about the doubleheader people would be seeing that night. We took a commercial break, and in the second segment, I flew solo.

"Welcome back. I need to take just a moment here to explain something that some of you may have wondered about in recent weeks. I'm dealing with something that millions of people have dealt with. Cancer. Specifically, follicular non-Hodgkin's lymphoma. The only reason I'm bringing my condition to your attention now is because the swelling of a lymph node here on the left side of my face has become noticeable. I was diagnosed two and a half years ago and have been having regular checkups since then.

"Through all of this time, I have had no symptoms. I've felt great and still do to this day. The plan my oncologist and I have settled on is to work the rest of the NBA season and play-offs, go to the beach with my wife, Cheryl, and

147

our four kids, and then start a treatment regimen in June, which will likely include chemotherapy. Then next season I'll come back to work, whether you like it or not. I draw much inspiration for what lies ahead from my mother, Lois, and my sister Dawn—both cancer survivors. As for my family, we will continue to do what we always do. We will trust God . . . period."

The outpouring of support and encouragement I received was staggering. NBA commissioner David Stern called the following day. The in-box of my computer's email was filled nonstop with well wishes and prayers from my Turner Sports family, friends I hadn't heard from in ages, and total strangers who had managed to get my email address. My bosses at the time, Turner Sports president David Levy and vice president Jeff Behnke, could not have been more compassionate, assuring me that they would be there for any needs my family might have and that there was no hurry for me to get back to work once my treatments began. "We just want you to get better, EJ. When you get back on the air, you get back on the air. We know you want to be back in the chair for opening night of the next NBA season, but there is no pressure on our end. We just want you better, no matter how long that takes."

And then there was the family at the Mexican restaurant in Dallas. Blackberry moment. I was there for the 2006 Western Conference Finals between the Mavericks and the Phoenix Suns and was now three weeks from the start of chemo. I had grabbed an early dinner on one of the nights there wasn't a game in Dallas and was waiting for the check. That's when a man walked away from the table where his family was sitting and over to mine. He said he watched the show regularly and knew what my upcoming summer included. Then he said, "We asked your waiter to bring us your check. It would be our pleasure to buy your dinner. Go get 'em."

Chemotherapy sessions, or infusions, can take a while. At least mine did. It really depends on what kind of chemo you're getting and how many drugs or antibodies are being used. I would be getting R-CHOP, each letter representing the various drugs used. I would list them here, but only a finalist in the national spelling bee would have a shot at correctly identifying them. For instance: "cyclophosphamide." Could I have the language of origin? Are there alternate spellings? Could you repeat the word? Is there an alternate pronunciation? Could you use it in a sentence? "Ernie's chemotherapy treatment included the drug cyclophosphamide." You get the idea.

My first infusion came in late June of 2006, and I was scheduled to have no fewer than six "cycles" (one infusion every three weeks) and possibly eight or nine depending on how well everything went. On a typical infusion day, I'd be sitting in a recliner by 9:00 a.m., headphones on, plugged into my iPod or the bedside television, and I'd be just one of the twenty or so patients watching bags of cancer-fighting drugs slowly drip . . . drip . . . drip into the tubing that ran from the infusion machines into ports that had been surgically implanted into our chests. Four bags of fluid were on the menu at each session, along with prednisone tablets, and I wouldn't walk out until 3:00 in the afternoon.

Most of the patients had a spouse, or another family member, or a friend sitting with them during the process. They'd be having conversations, or watching TV, or reading, or knitting, or working on their computers while the treatment was going on. I just wanted to be alone. Cheryl would drop me off in the morning and pick me up in the afternoon, sitting with me for the last half hour as the last of the drugs entered my system. She always said she would sit with me for the duration, but I always told her it wasn't necessary. She could take care of the kids or go to work. She didn't have to sit there for five or six hours and watch me sleep, or watch TV, or throw up. I'd heard all the stories about chemo and had read quite a bit about it. It was like the lab technician had said (yes, the one who had told me, "You may have cancer, but it doesn't have you"): "I don't know what you've heard, but the entertainment value of chemotherapy is really, really overrated." I appreciated him trying to lighten the mood whenever possible, because even though I had done my research, I had no idea exactly which of the nasty side effects I might experience.

If there's one thing I hate, as I would guess most of you do, it's throwing up. It had rarely happened to me; in fact, I could remember the five times it had happened—the locations are exact; the dates are in the ballpark.

1. Brattleboro, Vermont, while visiting my grandparents (1960)
2. Milwaukee, Wisconsin, in my pajamas (1962)
3. Atlanta, Georgia, when I had the flu (1968)
4. Philadelphia, Pennsylvania, after covering the Braves' season opener (1985)
5. Vancouver, British Columbia, the last time I would ever eat sea bass (1997)

No way I wanted Cheryl or anybody else to be on hand for number six if chemo was going to have that effect. And you know what? It never did. Not once in the course of all my treatments. That's not to say there weren't some difficult stretches.

I woke up that Saturday morning after my first chemo session the day before and felt . . . normal. I made sure I took my pills with breakfast, spent some time reading on the back patio, took a walk, and relaxed, and it was like any other day. And so was Sunday. Chemo novice that I was, I felt pretty good about how things were going, so good that I wanted to check with Dr. Heffner to make sure something had actually been in all those bags that was doing what it was supposed to be doing, because if I was supposed to be having any side effects, they weren't happening.

A few days later I could hardly get out of bed.

I had chills so bad in the middle of the night that I went to my closet and put on sweats and socks and a hoodie. This was July in Atlanta. Normally, those things had been stashed away for the summer. At 5:30 in the morning, I was shivering. Cheryl stuck a thermometer in my mouth. It read 103. She called Emory Hospital, and soon, with the sun just beginning to come up, my son Eric was driving me there. This was one of those times when you realize that even though just one person in the family *has* cancer, it *attacks* everybody. I knew this had to be hard for Eric—his dad in the front seat beside him, looking as sick as he had ever seen him.

When we got to the hospital, I was taken to a room where my vitals were taken, blood was drawn, and medication was given, and I actually began feeling coherent enough to ask when my son and I could go back home. The nurse looked at me with sort of a half smile and said, "Well, it won't be today. We'll have a room for you upstairs in just a minute."

My white cell count was low. Really low. White cells fight off infections, and I didn't have much defense. I would be in the hospital until my count was high enough. It would turn out to be five days, and the first few were spent virtually in isolation. When I was allowed to get out of bed and walk around, I was limited to a few laps around the hospital floor and was thrilled on day four to be let outside for a few minutes wearing a surgical mask.

Four days after being sent home, I was back at Emory for my second cycle of chemotherapy. To avoid a repeat of what had happened the first time, my doctor added another step to my regimen. Two days after every treatment, I would drive to the infusion center for a shot of a drug called Neulasta, which helps the body make white blood cells. That stuff is the bomb. And the great thing about it was that I would be in and out of the infusion center in ten minutes. While I was in there getting the shot, I witnessed the familiar scene—every recliner occupied by a cancer patient getting their treatment. By this time, I had become familiar with the nonverbal communication common to members of the cancer club. I would make eye contact with a man or a woman hooked up to the chemotherapy machinery and simply give a clenched fist. Some would return that sign, or just nod, or slowly blink to show the message had been received.

While from that second treatment on I tolerated chemo pretty well, there were days I didn't feel like doing much of anything but staking out a spot on the couch. I was able to work out on a fairly regular basis. When my hair started falling out, I took the initiative of shaving my head rather than going through a period of time looking like a stray dog with mange. I wore that hairless look like a badge of honor. I was in a fight, and in my mind, I was winning. There were certainly times when fear and doubt and anxiety came knocking at my door. I would simply say, "You can come in, but you're gonna have to hang out with faith, trust, and hope—and they're not gonna let you stay here long."

A couple things were troublesome, and I hesitate to even bring them up, because so many of the patients going through what I was had far worse stories to relate. Mealtimes were tricky, if not maddening. Cheryl would ask me what I felt like eating and would offer a few suggestions. She makes tremendous turkey, cheese, and tomato panini, and in the moment she would bring that up, I'd be all in. Then she'd bring it to the table, and the aroma, which under normal conditions would have my mouth watering, would make me gag. One Thursday morning, as I joined my buddies at Bible study, I ordered scrambled eggs, bacon, and grits—my staple. I couldn't even look at the plate when it was delivered and just apologized to the waitress and the group and drove home.

Then there were my eyebrows. I didn't have a problem with the bald look, and in time there wasn't a hair on my body, but not having eyebrows gave me kind of a mannequin quality I wasn't thrilled with. I could only chalk that up to vanity. But the good thing about looking in the mirror was this: the swelling in my face was quickly disappearing and I felt strong. I felt alive! The weeks went by with a third and fourth cycle in the books.

In mid-July, when I should have been sitting in the eighteenth tower calling the British Open at Royal Liverpool, I was in my Emory recliner watching the coverage on TNT, hearing Mike Tirico and the announcing crew send me their best. It meant the world. Just as it did in August when I had

153

to miss the PGA Championship in Chicago and Billy Andrade finished his second round with a share of the lead and concluded his post-round interview with some kind words about me and my cancer battle and how he looked forward to having me back in the tower at the PGA the following year.

At the same time, I was being encouraged by daily emails of support. If there's one thing I learned from that summer of 2006, it was the value of having friends hit the send button. You have no idea what it meant when I was having "one of those days," when nausea was trying to get the upper hand or I was simply exhausted, and then I'd see a list of emails to be read telling me to "hang in there," or "keep up the fight," or "our church prayed for you last Sunday." It was an inspirational shot of adrenaline.

So here's the deal. If you know somebody who's going through something—it doesn't have to be cancer; it can be any number of trials we all face from time to time—take a minute, write a note, and hit the send button. With that simple gesture, you can instantly provide a blackberry moment in the life of someone who's struggling.

Nobody understood the power of encouragement better than my sister Chris. She had been a longtime special education teacher who had retired and now had time to focus on endeavors that were much more than hobbies—animal rescue, gardening, and quilt making. She was not a runner, but in honor of my fight, she trained for one of the country's largest annual 10K (6.2 miles) runs, the Peachtree Road Race. She was one of more than forty thousand who took part on the Fourth of July, and she ran it with a shirt proclaiming that she was running for her brother. When my fiftieth birthday rolled around in August, she presented me with a beautiful quilt that I could take to treatment with me because I always asked for a blanket or two while I sat in the recliner. Sewn into that five-foot-by-five-foot masterpiece was the message "For every season there is a miracle."

My sixth, and potentially final, chemo cycle came on October 13, with the 2006–2007 NBA season set to start seventeen nights later. After more than three months, I had gotten to know the infusion staff at the Winship Cancer Institute very well. Often during those hours of treatment, when I wasn't reading, or listening to music, or watching those full bags of fluid gradually empty, I would just watch the nurses tend to other patients. What must that be like, I wondered, to wake up in the morning and head to a job where you deal on a daily basis with life and death, watching some patients improve and others decline? It takes a special person to do that, and I had nothing but the utmost respect for the jobs they did and the compassion they showed. They were angels in hospital scrubs and rubber gloves and surgical masks. All of that being said, I never wanted to see them again.

Tuesday, October 31—Halloween—was opening night of the NBA season with a doubleheader on TNT, and I was back in the host chair, sitting with my buddies Kenny and Charles, and now all of us were bald. I had no idea it was coming, but our remote crews who would televise the games from Miami and Los Angeles that night had done interviews with several players welcoming me back, and our studio production team had taken those clips and pieced them together. The video ended with Kobe Bryant saying that now with my bald head, "You're officially a brother." It was a special way to start the night.

The following morning, Wednesday, November 1, I was back at Winship for my latest scan, which would determine if the six cycles had done the trick or if I would be back in the infusion room two days later for another round of chemo. I would know in about twenty-four hours. So on Thursday, I was in my office by noon preparing for another TNT doubleheader, going through my usual game day routine of reading articles from various newspaper outlets around the league, updating my notes on the games played the previous night, and preparing some discussion points on the two games we would televise that night. And I waited for the phone to ring. And I waited. And I waited some more. At 4:00, I went down the hall for a production meeting led by our producer Tim Kiely. That took about a half hour, and when I got back to my office, I was hoping to see the blinking red light on my phone, indicating a message, hopefully from Dr. Heffner. No such luck. And then shortly after 6:00 the phone rang, and I recognized the number. This was it. I took a deep breath and picked up after the second ring.

"Ernie, this is Dr. Heffner. I know you're at work. Do you have a minute?"

"I've got whatever time you need."

"Well, I've got the results of your scan yesterday, and I have some good news. I know we talked about possibly having as many as eight or nine cycles of chemotherapy, but your scan came back clean. Your cancer is in remission. So don't worry about coming in tomorrow. You're done with chemo."

"Well, that *is* good news."

It was news I couldn't wait to share with my wife, so as soon as I'd hung up with Dr. Heffner, I called Cheryl at home.

A journey that had begun with tears back in August of 2003 was now ending that way over a telephone line.

After our call, still an hour or so from having to go on the air, I sat at my desk and reflected on what the last three unscripted years had been like. The fears, the anxiety, the constant wondering if I would be around for graduations and weddings and grandchildren. All those looks of concern on the faces of Eric and Maggie and Carmen and Michael. All those hours in the infusion recliner. All those messages from friends who had hit the send button. All those prayers I had said in times of stress when it was just me talking to the God who had created me, asking for strength and the peace that passes all understanding and for another badly needed dose of trust. And now it was over. I let an overwhelming sense of gratitude wash over me. God had gifted me with faith and family and friends, and I truly was the richest man in town.

12

I'm Good with That

I DON'T WANT TO SOUND CORNY HERE, or trite, or hokey, or banal, or hackneyed. (Sorry, I just got this new thesaurus and can't put it down.) But you hear folks talk about having this "new appreciation for life" or viewing "every day as a gift" after they've been through something that's been a life changer. Something like cancer. When I used to hear somebody say those things, I don't think I scoffed at them; I just couldn't quite grasp the concept. I felt I always had an appreciation for what I had—beautiful wife, great kids, fun job. But in the course of "doing life," sometimes that appreciation drifted into the background just a bit. If you've ever felt that life had basically become getting from point A to point B, I'm right there with you. You know what I'm talking about—you've probably heard yourself say it.

"Oh, I'm so slammed right now. I just need to get through Wednesday, and I'll relax."

"I'm just thinking that tomorrow afternoon at this time this will all be finished."

"This is our busiest time of the year. I'm just trying to make it to the end of the month."

"Oh, I wish I could fast-forward three weeks."

Well, here's the thing. After that whole health scare/cancer reality/chemo fun, I found that I really didn't want time to speed up. I didn't want to have self-imposed or oftentimes work-imposed deadlines dictate the rhythm of my life. Sure, they were going to be there—there's no eliminating them—but I was going to make a conscious effort to slow down, to stroll through the blackberry bramble and not miss anything. I was going to be present in the moment and not preoccupied with how busy things were *about* to become. So in that respect, I did gain a new appreciation for what every day might bring and was grateful to be given each and every one of them.

Dallas Willard said it best in a story related by John Ortberg in his book *Soul Keeping*: "Hurry is the great enemy of spiritual life in our day. You must ruthlessly eliminate hurry from your life."[2] Man, that's a good one. And the more I considered it, the more I realized that when I'm in a hurry, everything becomes about me. I'm cutting it close getting to the airport, and the TSA line is glacier-like. "Am I gonna miss my flight? What if I do and can't find another flight that gets me there when I need to be there?" Traffic on Interstate 85 between my home in Braselton and Atlanta is moving slower than the TSA line. "Will this put me behind in my prep for the game? Will this make me late for the meeting?"

You see, when I'm living my life trying to stay one second ahead of the deadline, I rush right past the person at the airport wearing that "Yes, I'm confused, but I'm trying not to look like it" expression as they try to figure out how to get from gate B31 to gate T18. When I'm not in a hurry to stay on my schedule, I have time to explain which escalator to get on, which train to board, and how many stops it'll be. Or even better, I just say, "Follow me. I'll getcha over there."

When I'm rushed and focused solely on my agenda, I drive right past the family of four broken down on the side of the road in ninety-five-degree heat. Only when I stop and admit that while I know nothing about automotive repair, I'd be happy to give them a lift to somebody who does and wind up paying for their car repairs and buying their lunch—*only then* can I feel I'm truly trying to fulfill a purpose greater than my own. Only when I learn they were coming back from the funeral of a relative hundreds of miles away when their car broke down do I start to think, "You know, there was a reason I left the house when I did and took the route I did."

These are matters in the spiritual realm, and as Dallas Willard said, "Hurry is the great enemy of spiritual life." I bring up instances like these not so you'll say, "Man, he is a great guy" but to point out that I stand in awe on a daily basis of the way God orchestrates life—how he connects the dots in ways I could never dream of if only I have the eyes to see and the heart to feel. And that's not me—that's how my Creator wired me.

This "nonbeliever" Cheryl Deluca-Johnson goes to Romania . . . and meets this orphan the nurse says is "no good" . . . and then calls her husband, Ernie, whose faith is dormant . . . and he says, despite what he and his wife had talked about, "Bring him home" . . . and this basketball coach from Indiana moves to Hoschton, Georgia, of all places . . . and puts this wheelchair-bound Romanian orphan on his basketball team . . . and in the process teaches kids at Mill Creek High School what it means to love. Sorry. That didn't just happen.

God did that.

I trust that.

I'm good with that.

In fact, I'm great with that.

And when this headstrong TV guy happens to get information about a nondenominational church in Lawrenceville, Georgia . . . and then meets the pastor . . . and they say a prayer at lunch . . . and Jesus becomes central in his life . . . and cancer blindsides him . . . and he doesn't fight it alone but vows to "trust God . . . period" . . . and comes out the other side with his cancer in remission . . . and then six months later finds himself standing in front of TV's best at the Sports Emmy Awards in New York . . . and he's accepting the Emmy for best studio host . . . and in his speech he says that "going through cancer taught him that God sometimes whispers and sometimes shouts that his way is better than my way" . . . Sorry. That series of events didn't just happen.

God did that too.

I'm good with that.

In fact, I'm great with that.

In 2011, I'm watching my eighty-seven-year-old father, my best man, my best friend, my mentor, my role model wasting away from congestive heart failure and the early stages of Alzheimer's. And I'm asking God, as if he needs my permission, to take him, to ease his suffering. And one more thing . . . let me be there when it's time. On the morning of August 12, he's been in hospice care for a week, and I stop by to see him on my way to the Atlanta Athletic Club, where the 2011 PGA Championship is being played, and I'm anchoring TNT's coverage. And we sit, and I talk, and I'm hoping he can hear me. And I tell him for the millionth time how much I love him and then head to the golf course to work. The slow pace of play that day in round two means we stay on the air longer than expected, about twenty minutes past what was to be our 7:00 p.m. sign-off. The round completed, I leave the TV compound as quickly as I can, and while making the twenty-minute drive to the facility called Embracing Hospice, my phone rings, and my brother-in-law Jacky Cheek is on the other end telling me to hurry. I enter the room to find my mother sitting in the corner. She rises and hugs me. Her eyes are filled with tears.

"Oh, Ernie."

And I see my father, mouth open, eyes closed, lifeless. I got there too late.

For the next five minutes, I just hug him and sob. His pain is gone. Mine is intense. I lost the most important figure in my life, and I was not there to hold his hand or whisper "I love you" when it happened. What if we hadn't had to stay on the air past 7:00? Could I have made it in time? To this day I have struggled with that question, which remains unanswered. I have beaten myself up over it. But at the same time, when I take myself out of the equation, which is vital if not difficult to do, I realize that my mother, Lois, my dad's wife of more than sixty years, was there for that moment, and I guess that's the way it was supposed to play out. And again I strive to trust God . . . period . . . that those final moments of my father's earthly life played out exactly as they were designed.

And only God knows that.

And while it's taken a long, long time, I'm good with that. In fact, I'm great with that.

Just under one month later, Saturday, September 10, 2011, I packed an overnight bag for a trip to Milwaukee, where the next day I would call the baseball game between the Milwaukee Brewers and the Philadelphia Phillies as part of our Sunday package on TBS. I had a 2:00 flight that afternoon and would swing by the Georgia Dome in downtown Atlanta to watch my daughter Carmen play in the Georgia State marching band before the GSU Panthers played football. We always joked that folks could tell Carmen was adopted because her musical talents certainly didn't come from anybody in our family. She could play the guitar, the piano, the flute, and the piccolo and was now a member of the Georgia State drum line.

While I was at the dome I got a call from Cheryl telling me that Michael was sick, was having trouble breathing, and we talked about whether he needed to be taken to the hospital. I made calls to the hospital in north Atlanta that was across the street from Michael's respiratory specialist and arranged for him to be taken there. I changed my 2:00 flight to 6:00 and met Cheryl and Michael at the hospital. Michael was twenty-three now and was struggling. It was pneumonia, and when you have muscular dystrophy, that's major. He doesn't have the strength to clear his lungs like we do.

The doctor arranged for Michael to be admitted, and Cheryl told me that with things under control I should go to the airport for my 6:00 flight. I would be back home in just over twenty-four hours after the Sunday game in Milwaukee. Once I got to Milwaukee, I checked in with Cheryl a couple times, and she told me Michael was resting comfortably and was in better shape than when I'd left him that afternoon.

When I'm doing weekend baseball, I have a Saturday night/Sunday morning routine. I fill in some of the scorebook the night before, listing the umpires, the pitchers in each team's bullpen, and various notes on each team. In the morning, after the league stats have all been updated following Saturday night's game, I go through about fifteen statistical categories and jot down the numbers relevant to the game we're televising. To get that work done, I normally set my alarm for 6:00 a.m. on Sunday and am on my way to the ballpark by 9:00 for a 1:00 first pitch. But on that Sunday, September 11, before my alarm had a chance to go off, my phone rang, and Cheryl was frantic. When the nurse had checked on Michael early that morning in Atlanta, he had been unresponsive. *Code blue* is a term used when a patient requires immediate attention to be revived. Michael had coded, and a resuscitation team had been called. They were using paddles—defibrillators—to try to keep him alive. Cheryl handed the phone to the doctor who was standing next to her and asking if she had our permission to intubate, to insert a breathing tube in Michael's trachea.

"Is this an absolute necessity? What if we don't?"

"Your son will die, Mr. Johnson."

"Then you do everything you have to do."

I tried to calm Cheryl. She had seen it all happen—Michael lying perfectly still, his fingers blue, the alarm alerting the team, the furious code blue activity—before a nurse had ushered her into the hallway. I knew there was nothing I could say that would erase those images.

Our travel department put me on the first flight out of Milwaukee, and I walked into the intensive care unit at 2:00

that afternoon. Michael was hooked up to more machines than I cared to count. My daughter Carmen says I just stood there saying, "Oh, Michael . . . Michael . . . Michael," but I remember none of that. I just remember a feeling of utter helplessness. The rest of the family had been there for hours, but now I would see them for the first time as Cheryl and I walked into the waiting room. We had all just been through a tough stretch, losing my dad the month before.

My mother voiced exactly what I was thinking. "This can't be happening. It's just too soon."

Michael was in the ICU for two weeks. The breathing tube they'd inserted on that frantic Sunday morning was in the next few days replaced by what would be a permanent fixture. He'd had a tracheotomy, and so now clear plastic tubing extended from his windpipe and was hooked to a ventilator at his bedside. That machine would allow Michael to breathe, and we were told that while sometimes that can be a temporary thing, Michael would never come off the vent. After two weeks, doctors told us Michael had reached the point that he could be taken out of intensive care but still needed to be hospitalized, and they recommended a facility that specialized in long-term acute care.

On September 23, he was taken by ambulance about sixty-five miles to Landmark Hospital in Athens. Michael may not be able to communicate as well as the rest of us and can't tell us point-blank that "it hurts here, right around my third rib, when I inhale" or "my lower back hurts when the bed is reclined at that angle," and that certainly can make caring for him challenging, but he is a fighter. We had no idea how long this next hospital stay would last or if it would even end with Michael going home with us. All we knew was this: we would be with him every day, and that meant rather than hitting the road to call the American League Division and Championship series on TBS, I'd be doing what every other baseball fan would be doing—watching them on TV. But I'd be watching from Michael's hospital room.

Cheryl and I took turns staying overnight, with our oldest daughter, Maggie, taking a night or two as well, sleeping in a bedside recliner. *Sleeping* is probably not an accurate term. With nurses making numerous visits in the wee hours to administer breathing treatments, or take vital signs, or draw blood, we did more "resting" than sleeping. The overnight settings on Michael's ventilator made it impossible for him to speak, so if he needed to get our attention in the middle of the night, he would make sounds, hoping we'd notice. And then we would try to read his lips. "Rub back." . . . "Go pee." . . . "Muscle hurts." . . . "Love you too."

So let me try to give you a snapshot of where we were. There was the *obvious* stuff. There was a machine—the vent—that allowed Michael to breathe. There was a feeding tube hanging from his stomach through which he got liquid meals. There were IV lines that led to bags of antibiotics hanging from IV poles. And there were various beeps and tones coming from his machines, some of which were just normal, routine sounds, and some of which sent a nurse double time into the room.

What we couldn't see, and what Dr. Tony Sagel was working tirelessly to determine, was why Michael couldn't shake a series of infections. He was experiencing FUOs—fevers of unknown origin. There were early signs of sepsis, a frightening condition in which bloodstream infections spread through the body and damage the internal organs. The only times

Michael left his bed for three weeks was when he was lifted out of it and placed on an ambulance stretcher to be taken down the street to Athens Regional Hospital.

On one trip, he was given a CT scan of his spine, and on another, he had an electrocardiogram (EKG) to see if there was an infection of his heart valves. Then there was the procedure called a thoracentesis. Fluid had built up between Michael's chest wall and lungs. Nurses had to hold him in a seated position because he couldn't support himself. Dr. Hugh Jenkins inserted a tube into Michael's right side just below his rib cage. Normally, there is a tablespoon of fluid in that area. Dr. Jenkins drained two liters. Not two teaspoons, or two tablespoons, or two cups—two liters. Tell me, where are the blackberry moments when you're watching your son go through this? Sometimes you find them in a post-op conversation.

"How'd it go, Dr. Jenkins?"

"It went well. We drained two liters at this point, and the tube is still in place, so we'll likely get more out of there when he's back at Landmark this afternoon."

"And he did okay? Is he hurting?"

"Well, it's not the most comfortable procedure, and given that he has MD, we had to hold him really steady, but he did just fine. But you know what he said when we were finished?"

"I don't, but just taking a shot, I'm sure it had something to do with what you or the nurses drive."

"No, we went through that before we started. When we were finished and got him back on the bed, he looked at me and whispered, 'Good job.' That's a pretty special young man."

"Can't argue with you there."

Back to Dr. Tony Sagel for a moment. He saved Michael's life. He was the one who in time, through a frustrating and sometimes maddening process of trial and error, doggedly tracked down the source of Michael's infections and subsequent fevers. There were times my phone would ring, and it would be Dr. Sagel.

"Hey, you know that culture we took from Michael this morning? Came back negative. But don't worry. I've got another idea on what might be causing this. We'll get there."

He was right; we did get there. Four weeks into Michael's stay at Landmark, the source of the infections was discovered, the medicine he needed was pumped into his veins, and the color returned to his face. Michael started to become Michael again. We were able to get him out of bed and into his wheelchair, and with his ventilator and a few other machines in tow, he was allowed to go outside for an hour or two to get some fresh air. As his fifth week at Landmark began, Cheryl and Maggie and I commenced a crash course on how the ventilator operated, what every alarm meant, how to work the suction machine to clear his lungs, how to connect the oxygen tanks and adjust how much he needed, how to use the machine that measured the oxygen saturation of his blood and his heart rate. He had a lot of gear.

Michael's favorite nurse, Brooke Stoyle, or Brookie, as he called her, taught us how to perform daily trach care—how to quickly and efficiently (a matter of seconds) disconnect Michael from his ventilator to change the inner cannula, the tube that's inserted into his trachea. We had all of the equipment we'd need to turn Michael's bedroom at home into a hospital room and were required to have a natural gas–powered generator installed at the house that would immediately kick in if we ever lost power so his equipment wouldn't be affected. By the end of the fifth week, on October 27, Dr. Sagel told us the words we were dying to hear but had often doubted we ever would.

"You can take Michael home."

Now the nursing training we'd received in Athens would be put to the test at home in Braselton. It would be a few weeks before we were able to finalize with our insurance company the details of overnight nursing coverage. In time, we would have a nurse every night from 10:00 p.m. until 10:00 the next morning. But in those early weeks, it was Cheryl and Maggie and me. It's one thing to hear a machine's alarm go off at 3:00 in the morning at Landmark. You just ring for the nurse to come in. Now for the time being, *we* were the nurses.

And we were doing okay.

I'm underselling that.

Let me put humility aside here for a second.

We were pretty darn good.

And if we needed any validation in that regard, we got it, unsolicited from Michael's new pulmonologist, Dr. Craig Brown, who saw him once a month and changed the entire trach apparatus every other month. He would check Michael out in his office and look us in the eye and inspire us.

"You folks are doing an incredible job. Keep it up. He looks great. His lungs sound great. Keep doing what you're doing."

You can't put a value on feedback like that or on the text message with his name on it simply asking, "How's our boy feeling today? Did we knock out that little fever from Tuesday? Just wanted to check in."

This unscripted phase of Michael's journey had brought with it a lot more equipment and a lot more responsibility, but we weren't running from it or cursing it. We were embracing it. In the course of what was a difficult situation, each day bringing a new challenge, Cheryl and I had a deep appreciation for what was required of me as a father and Cheryl as a mother. When you're doing *everything* for a young man who doesn't have the strength to do *anything* on his own, a powerful essence of servanthood becomes ingrained. When you wake up in the morning and suction the mucus from your son's lungs, and you position his body in a sling attached to a ceiling-mounted lift system, and you take him to the bathroom and wash him and shave him and dress him, and you get him into his wheelchair, all the while making sure that every machine is correctly set, it's downright impossible to think about yourself. I need that. It forces me to wake up each morning with the attitude "What can I do for you?" not "What can you do for me?" In its own way, it provides a daily blackberry moment.

Michael had lost a lot of weight in the hospital—thirty-seven pounds. He hadn't eaten solid food since September 9, and now it was the day before Thanksgiving, November 23, and we were in midtown Atlanta for a swallow test to see if Michael, now permanently attached to a ventilator and with the continued weakening of his muscles because of MD, was capable of swallowing solid food without choking.

It was a fascinating test actually. He was given applesauce and saltine crackers and peanut butter, all coated with dye, and somehow we could watch on a monitor as he chewed and swallowed. And I'll be doggone if he didn't pass that test. We got the go-ahead to start him the next day on soft, moist foods that would be easy to handle, and we could progress from there.

Where are the blackberry moments when you deal with a life-and-death situation like the one Michael had been through? Well, you find them when you're gathered around a Thanksgiving table in 2011. This kid who had coded, who was now on life support but was finally home, wasn't having his meal poured from a can through a feeding tube. He was smiling and eagerly awaiting the next spoonful of stuffing, drenched in gravy, on what will forever be our most unforgettable and gratitude-filled Thanksgiving Day. And you know what?

God did that.

I'm good with that.

In fact, I'm great with that.

13

Father of the Bride . . . and the Groom

You won't find a member of the Johnson family who was sorry to see 2011 end. To say that was a tough year is sort of like saying Oprah likes a slice of bread occasionally.

You also won't find a member of the Johnson family who will forget 2012, specifically the summer of that year, when the two oldest Johnson kids got married. Not to each other. We actually had three wedding ceremonies in a span of sixty-four days. I know the math doesn't work—two kids, three ceremonies—but hey, we've always taken a rather unique route, and this was no different.

All right, you dads with unmarried girls out there, buckle up. We're talking about that season of life when you watch your firstborn daughter discover the man of her dreams.

And it's not you.

In the case of my daughter Maggie, it was Dustin Pruitt. They had gone to the same high school but weren't high school sweethearts by any means—it's not one of those stories. They had stayed in touch during their college years and then in time reconnected, and now their relationship had gotten to the serious point. Cheryl had told me she had the feeling that one of these days Dustin would come to me with his desire to marry my daughter, and take care of her, and be the best husband of all time. I was really looking forward to that. I wanted her to marry him.

Dustin's a good guy—bright kid, civil engineer, has definite plans on where he sees his life going. I rarely called him Dustin to be honest. I shortened it to D. "Hey, give me a hand with this ladder, will ya, D?" "Whoa! Nice putt, D." And then I lengthened that to D-Train for no good reason, and that's what I called him. "Hey, when are you gonna ask if you can marry my daughter, D-Train?" In short, he is just the kind of guy you *want* asking for your daughter's hand in marriage.

So now I was just waiting to see how he would go about this. When he and Maggie would be over at the house, I would be halfway expecting him to ask if we could step outside for a second to talk. Or I'd wander out to the back patio where he was building a fire in our outdoor fireplace, and it would be just the two of us, and the time would be perfect for the conversation.

"Ern, I got a question."

"Yeah, D-Train, whatcha got?"

"Where'd you get this firewood? It catches really fast."

Turns out the best time to ask me about marrying my daughter was a cool Sunday evening that winter as I was rolling our trash cans to the street for the Monday pickup. Really. I had taken one down to the curb and turned around to go get the other, and Dustin . . . uh . . . D-Train was standing in the middle of the driveway. This didn't take long, and it had nothing to do with firewood.

"What's up, D-Train?"

"Well, I think you have a pretty good idea how I feel about Maggie. I love her and want her to be my wife, and I need you to know that. Not exactly sure how I'm going to propose or when it will happen, but it'll be soon."

"Well, you know how much Cheryl and I love you, Dustin. We couldn't ask for a better son-in-law."

We sealed the deal with the combination handshake and man hug. It works for everything. A few weeks later Dustin proposed, and Maggie said yes.

And now, dads, here comes the tough part. Preparing yourself for that day, which at this point is still months away, when you will walk your daughter down the aisle and hope you do not ruin the moment by being a total sniffling, boo-hooing mess. As I've already told you, the film *Father of the Bride* wrecks me. There is one scene in particular when Steve Martin (the dad) and Kimberly Williams-Paisley (his daughter) are playing basketball in the driveway, and he sees her as a child and then as a teenager, and now she's engaged, and well, it just turns me into the mess I don't want to be when her wedding day arrives.

And now as we're preparing for a June wedding, I'm Steve Martin times a thousand. I'm picturing Maggie in her softball uniform as a five-year-old, and I'm seeing her as a middle school cheerleader, and then suddenly she is a beautiful high school senior with an adorable personality. And I'm thinking about those times when I had to deal with the emotions of a teenage girl, replaying those moments of high school crisis when I wasn't sure if the approach I took would make

175

me a lifetime pal or a temporary—at least I hoped it was a temporary—adversary.

Like the time she tried out for the middle school cheerleading squad and made it to the final cut. She was a wreck during the final week of tryouts, and I tried to calm her nerves by telling her what my dad had taught me about effort: "Once you've done your best, to heck with it." I gave her a small card I'd bought one day that simply read, "Relax. God's in charge." That week, as her anxiety grew, I gave her a hug and said, "Hey, read the card." When the cheerleading squad was selected, the names were posted on the wall of the gymnasium. Maggie and her friends crowded around the list, and there were shrieks of delight and lots of hugging and jumping around . . . for those who had made it. Maggie's name wasn't on the list. Not much a dad can do at that point but offer a shoulder to cry on and hopefully an encouraging word or two that will somehow ease the pain. And remind her to "read the card." Years later I was still using that, to the point that she would finish the sentence I started when she was going through a tough time.

"Oh, and one more thing, Mags . . ."

"I know, Dad. Read the card."

Neither Cheryl nor I wanted our kids to view us as helicopter parents. You know, parents who fly in and swoop down to rescue their kids from trouble. That's not the way we were brought up. My dad and mom always stressed taking personal responsibility. Maggie was a good student, but one year she was struggling with a high school honors math class. That comes from my side of the gene pool, because her mom's a wiz. Maggie was relieved to escape with a C one semester, but she wasn't so lucky the next. She was on the verge of failing the course, which would mean summer school. When I picked her up from school on the last day, she was frantic.

"Dad, you've gotta come inside and talk to my math teacher. She's gonna fail me. Can you do something?"

I did something. I walked into the classroom where the teacher was gathering her things and ready to call it a school year. She showed me her grade book and Maggie's scores on various tests and projects. The numbers didn't lie. Her average was sixty-eight. I thanked the teacher and walked into the hallway where Maggie was waiting.

"Well, Dad?"

"You've got a sixty-eight. Enjoy summer school." (I didn't tell her to "read the card" that time.)

Maggie ended up taking that summer school course online. To add to the learning experience, Cheryl, much to her credit, suggested that Maggie use the money she was earning babysitting for a neighbor to pay for the course. The final exam had to be taken in person, and here's where a painful teenage episode for our oldest daughter took a rather serendipitous turn.

On the day of the final, we walked into the lobby of the high school not knowing in which room the test would take place. A few other students were milling around, and Maggie asked one if he knew which room she needed to be in. He wasn't there for the test but had just dropped off a buddy who was, and he pointed down the hall. That helpful young man was a straight-A student named Dustin Pruitt, and that was the first time he and Maggie met. Now, years later, they were about to become husband and wife. True story.

So now here she is, a teacher in the making, about to embark on this whole new chapter with Dustin, the man of her dreams. Call me a lunatic, but the night before the wedding I ordered *Father of the Bride* on pay-per-view. Here was my rationale. If I could get through the movie this time without turning to mush, then maybe I'd turned the corner. Maybe I could handle what the next afternoon was going to be like. It didn't work. The same scenes that always got to me got to me again, but I was truly feeling like one blessed man. Maggie was all grown up now. In less than twenty-four hours, she'd be a wife, and I was thrilled for her. But there was also this melancholy side of me.

Dads who have been there and done that know what I'm talking about, and part of that feeling came from the knowledge that I couldn't ask my dad how he had gotten through it with my sisters, Dawn and Chris. He was gone, but to Maggie's credit, he wouldn't be forgotten when it came time for her special day. When my father had died the summer before, the Atlanta Braves had honored his memory by wearing patches on their uniforms for the remainder of the season. They were white with blue trim with "Ernie" stitched at the top, and below that was a baseball glove with a microphone in the pocket. Bill Acree, who was a fixture with the organization for the better part of fifty years and made all the team's travel arrangements as well as ran the clubhouse, had made sure that our family had all the patches we might need. On Maggie's wedding day, all the bouquets were bound at the bottom with those "Ernie" patches. Such a nice touch.

Technically, I wouldn't be walking Maggie *down the aisle* on June 30, 2012. I would be walking her from the front door of our house onto a stone path that led to a shaded patio area in the woods near our front yard. Cheryl had designed the area several years earlier as one of those places we could sit and watch the sun set through the trees while birds swooped in for dinner at the feeder, and often we would just sit there and unpack the day. We have areas in both the front and the back of our house for that very purpose and have found that in the busyness of our lives, those spots provide at least a temporary refuge where we can rest, or read, or pray, or listen to the wind, or watch a mama bird feed her screeching babies, or have heart-to-heart conversations, or talk about nothing in particular. They may not sound like much, but for us, these areas have been date night destinations where much of the decision-making in our lives has taken place.

Guys, here's a word of unsolicited advice: Date nights don't have to involve dinner reservations or movie tickets. They just need to be times when you're intentional about spending time with your wife. They can be a night on the town or an hour in the backyard. The key is that your attention is focused on one thing: your bride. Cheryl and I discovered this out of necessity really, because with Michael needing constant monitoring, we couldn't always leave the house. One of the kids could keep an eye on him, or we'd take one of those tiny video and audio monitors to the patio with us so we could hear if an alarm went off and could walk inside and respond. But this was time just for us, and after thirty-four years of marriage, I can say without hesitation you have to make time for that.

Years before she got engaged, Maggie had told us that one day she would be married in that front yard patio underneath the towering trees that gave relief from the Georgia sun. And now it was going to happen. And it was going to happen on *the* hottest day of 2012 in Atlanta. I'm not exaggerating. You can look it up: 104 degrees in Atlanta; 107 at our house in Braselton. But on the patio in the shade, I swear it didn't feel like more than 105. As if I needed another reason to sweat.

So how did it go? It was perfect. For one thing, nobody succumbed to heat exhaustion, and for another, I was actually able to feel my legs as I walked Maggie to the patio. And the smile I couldn't keep from my face wasn't forced—I just couldn't help it. I wasn't trying to act like I had it all together at this long-awaited moment. I actually did. I'll admit to a tear or two as I kissed Maggie's cheek and walked to my seat next to Cheryl, but I avoided the YouTube-worthy meltdown I had feared. Maggie and Dustin exchanged vows, everybody cheered, we took sixteen thousand pictures, and then we drove to the reception, where I would have one more blackberry moment with my baby girl. (Yes, she'll always be that.) We danced to one of Maggie's favorite songs, "Little Miss Magic" by Jimmy Buffett.

> Constantly amazed by the blades of the fan on the
>   ceiling.
> The clever little glances she gives me can't help but
>   be appealing.
> She loves to ride into town with the top down,
> Feel that warm breeze on her gentle skin.
> She is my next of kin.
> I see a little more of me every day.
> I catch a little more moustache turning gray.
> Your mother is the only other woman for me.
> Little Miss Magic, whatcha gonna be?
> Sometimes I catch her dreamin' and wonder where
>   that little mind meanders.

Is she strollin' along the shore or cruisin' o'er the
    broad savannah.
I know someday she'll learn to make up her own
    rhymes,
Someday she's gonna learn how to fly.
Oh, that I won't deny. . . .
I see a little more of me every day.
I feel a little more moustache turning gray.
Your mother's still the only other woman for me.
Little Miss Magic, whatcha gonna be?
Little Miss Magic, whatcha gonna be?
Little Miss Magic, just can't wait to see.[3]

The weddings we had that summer came after proposals delivered one night apart in February, something neither
groom-to-be had planned. It was a Wednesday night when
Dustin proposed to Maggie. Late that night the phone rang,
and it was our twenty-seven-year-old son, Eric. He had just
gotten off work at 11:30 after doing the graphics on NBA-TV.

"Hey, Dad, isn't it great about Mags and D-Train?"

"Yeah, we're all thrilled."

"Well, I've got a problem. I was planning to propose to
Quynh [pronounced Quinn] tomorrow night. How can I
do that now that Dustin just did? I mean, isn't this going to
be awkward—two proposals in two nights? Isn't it going to
seem strange or that I'm just doing this now because Maggie
and Dustin did? What am I going to do?"

"Eric, calm down a second. Take a deep breath. Do you
love Quynh?"

"Absolutely, Dad."

"Well . . . it's easy. Don't worry about who asked who, and when, and all that stuff. You guys are in love. You've made your decision. You're a wonderful couple. Your mom is going to be so excited. I'm proud of you, Eric. Go get 'em, kid."

"Thanks, Dad. I love you."

"Love you too, E. Now hang on. Your mom wants to talk to you."

Cheryl and Eric had one of those "Mom talking to her firstborn child about his imminent marriage proposal" conversations that left them both wading in their own tears. And the next night Quynh said yes.

Just as I was thrilled with the idea of Dustin as a son-in-law, I was equally enthralled with the idea of Quynh Truong as a daughter-in-law. Her story is fascinating. She was born in Vietnam in 1987. Her father, Dinh, fought with the South alongside United States forces in the Vietnam War. In 1975, after the fall of Saigon signaled the end of that brutal twenty-year war, the North Vietnamese imprisoned over one million supporters of the South in so-called reeducation camps. Dinh spent the next six years of his life in one of those camps, where mistreatment was the norm. Only after the first three years was he occasionally allowed visitors. In time, those camps were closed, and Dinh was released.

In 1991, he and his wife, Mang, brought their family, including eight-year-old son, Tuoc, and four-year-old daughter, Quynh, to California. Mang gave birth to another son, Alan, and eventually, the Truong family relocated to Georgia. Quynh was actually a high school classmate of Maggie's. That's how Eric got to know her, but it would be a few years before they started dating. Once they started, Eric had no chance. Quynh is delightful, fun-loving, and brilliant. She got her law degree from the University of South Carolina and is a practicing attorney in Atlanta. They would be married two months after Dustin and Maggie's wedding, on August 31 *and* September 1. Remember I said we had three weddings that summer. One for Maggie and two for Eric—the traditional American wedding on Friday night and the traditional Vietnamese ceremony the following morning.

The fact that Eric chose me to be his best man was special beyond words. My father had been mine back in 1982, and now, thirty years later, I would stand with my son as he exchanged vows with Quynh. Back in 1982, I hadn't known exactly what kind of gift to give my best man. It had to be something of significance that spoke of the love and respect I had for my father, and I wanted it to be something he could use. A watch? A money clip? No. A beer mug? Oh, now we're talkin'. I loved having a cold one with my dad while watching a ball game on TV, or after a day of yard work, or after a round of golf while we added up astronomical scores. So I found this big, heavy pewter mug in a gift store, and I had it engraved.

> *My Best Man*
> *My Best Friend*
> *August 21, 1982*

Fast-forward thirty years and ten days. We're at a beautiful wedding venue in Norcross, Georgia, called the Atrium, where everything is set for the outdoor ceremony on a perfect summer evening.

Eric is busying himself helping members of the wedding party with their bow ties, making sure their suits, which had been made by Quynh's aunt in Vietnam, look just right, and taking pictures with his groomsmen. When I'm not part of the picture taking, I'm just watching from a distance—and remembering. I'm remembering the day he was born a few weeks earlier than he was supposed to be. I'm thinking about his one season of soccer before the family tradition of baseball took hold of him. I'm thinking about all the days I anxiously watched him strike out hitters and the day I watched him drill a pitch into the trees beyond the right field fence at Collins Hill Park. And I see him pushing a stroller that holds his new brother fresh from a Romanian orphanage, and I see him volunteering at the muscular dystrophy camp as a teenager who doesn't need to be taught that there is value in everybody no matter their physical limitations.

And I'm thinking about more recent times, like when he went with me to the PGA Championship as a freelance runner working twelve-hour days doing whatever duty he was asked. And I remember an established crew member stopping me at the TV compound one morning to relate one of those stories that just makes you feel good as a dad.

"Ernie, is that your son Eric I had a chance to work with the other day?"

"Yeah, it probably was. He's had a great time. Long hours but great experience. Why do you ask?"

"Well, I've been doing this a long time and have had a lot of sons of announcers assigned to help me, but yours is different. The first thing most of these kids tell me is, 'My dad is so-and-so,' as if to put me on notice that I better take it easy on them or they'll tell their dad. I didn't know Eric was your son for four days until I asked somebody who this guy was. What a worker. You should be really proud. He gets it."

"Well, you just made my day."

These moments of reflection are interrupted by the sound of Eric's voice. We're thirty minutes from the start of the ceremony when he asks me to go inside to the groom's room. This kid—who had the "Ernie" patch sewn into the lining of our suit jackets—and I sit there and lock eyes, and his eyes are already getting misty as he simply thanks me for a lifetime of doing what dads do. Teaching, disciplining, modeling, molding, encouraging, hoping, praying. And I tell Eric that anything I learned about all that came from my dad, his grandfather, the right-hander, Poppy, Big Guy. Eric reaches behind the table where we are sitting and pulls out a box, which he hands to me. My hands are shaking as I open it, remove a few sheets of tissue paper, and find an engraved pewter beer mug. And in that moment, I am as speechless as my own father had been thirty years earlier.

My Best Man
My Best Friend
August 31, 2012

Whatever you think that scene looked like as I read that engraving and looked at my son, well, go with it. No way I can describe it. Won't even try. That evening I stood shoulder to shoulder with my firstborn son, now a grown man, making Quynh Truong his bride, and wondered if anything could make a dad feel prouder. The next day came close.

The Johnson family was now venturing into uncharted waters of Vietnamese tradition, ceremony, and wardrobe. I'm just guessing here, but if I asked for a show of hands from all those men who have worn an áo dài (pronounced

OW-yigh), I'm fairly certain we're talking low single digits. An áo dài is a head-to-toe silk robe. Mine was gold with a brown floral pattern. To complete the ensemble was a circular hat, hollowed out in the middle. I'll be the first to say it. I looked awesome—I mean, awkward. Cheryl did look stunning in hers—white silk pants with a flowing blue top. I do believe that Eric and I were wearing the biggest áo dàis ever made. No one on Quynh's side of the family is taller than five foot eight. My son and I are in the six-foot-two range. We were easy to spot that day, standing above the crowd, as Dinh and Mang hosted the ceremony at their house.

I understood very little (translated nothing) of what was being spoken in Vietnamese, though when a gesture was made in my direction and the name Ernie was spoken, I gave a little wave and a smile and then shot a quick glance at Eric to make sure I hadn't ruined the day. The ceremony was solemn and highlighted by some of the most heart-melting looks exchanged between Quynh and her parents. I'll never forget those. I guess they grow blackberries in Vietnam too.

When the ceremony was over, a day-long party ensued. The first few hours consisted of an early afternoon feast, which featured as the main course a whole roasted pig, and there was a variety of side dishes I could not pronounce but was game to try. Only one word could describe it—*delicious*—and we were just warming up. The evening brought another full-blown celebration at a nearby Vietnamese restaurant. The image of that night that I will never forget is of Eric and Quynh making the rounds at each and every table, where their union was toasted. In particular, I remember the stop made at Dinh's table, where he and his army buddies were gathered. They had been through hell together and were now savoring just a slice of heaven.

Once again I can't come up with words to describe the pride I felt for my son. You see, in Vietnamese culture, it's pretty much expected that your daughter will marry a man who has those same bloodlines. Eric obviously didn't fit that bill, but he had won them over by simply "being himself"—my father's lifelong advice again coming to the forefront. The Truong family had seen a man of integrity, a man of loyalty, a man intent on being the best husband they could imagine for their one and only daughter, and they had accepted him. It was a snapshot that proved once again that of all the forces of nature, love is by far the most powerful.

14

You Know 'Em
When You See 'Em

ONE OF THE GREAT THINGS about a blackberry moment is that you won't find it in any dictionary anywhere. It's a Johnson family thing and thus open to any definition we choose to come up with. So if the folks at Merriam-Webster or Funk and Wagnalls were to give me space, I guess the entry would look like this:

blackberry moment *n*

1. an unpredictable moment that makes life extraordinary
2. an unforeseen moment that catches you off guard and marks you forever
3. a moment so sweet that you savor the taste for a lifetime
4. a moment when God winks and you can swear you hear him whisper, "That's what I'm talkin' about."

We are surrounded by moments that fit these descriptions. It's not as if they come along so rarely that if we miss one, we'll never get the chance again. We've all heard the local weatherman finish his forecast by saying, "If you look into the eastern sky between 11:14 and 11:43 tonight, you'll see something that happens only once every 231 years." Blackberry moments aren't like that. And for the most part, they can't be predicted. They just happen. And hopefully, you've got a front-row seat to watch them. But here's the thing— you have to be present, and you have to be on the lookout, because they can pop up at any time, any place. And they have the power to change your perspective and in the process change your life . . . or somebody else's.

The National Academy of Television Arts & Sciences hosts the Sports Emmy Awards every spring. In the category of outstanding sports personality—studio host Bob Costas has been the gold standard for more than two decades. I have long maintained that the honor should be renamed the Costas. The guy has won seventeen of them in a twenty-three-year span. I've been fortunate enough to earn nine nominations in that category and to win it three times. And that third, in May 2015, was a blackberry. But not for me.

Among the five nominees that year was the popular Stuart Scott of ESPN, who in the course of eight years had battled cancer valiantly until it claimed his life in January 2015. It was safe to say that on Emmy night that year, the five other nominees in the category—Costas, Matt Vasgersian of MLB Network, Keith Olbermann of ESPN 2, Rich Eisen of NFL Network, and I—expected that when the winner was announced, Stuart Scott's name would be called, and his two daughters, Taelor and Sydni, would walk to the stage and accept the Emmy for their late father. We all knew it, and so did every other person in the ballroom filled with TV types from across the country.

Tom Verducci, the Emmy Award–winning reporter for MLB Network and Fox Sports, presented the night's final award. He opened the envelope and said, "And the Emmy goes to Ernie Johnson, TNT." Cheryl was with me in New York. We heard it but couldn't quite believe it. In fact, I had told her beforehand that surely Stuart would win and it would be a special moment to hear his daughters' acceptance speech. I had also vowed to myself that if I were ever lucky enough to win another Emmy, I would bring my wife onstage with me and salute her in front of the crowd for all she had meant to me throughout the years, for all the sacrifices she had made while putting up with my crazy schedule, and for holding our family together in the midst of all that. Now I had the opportunity to do so, but at the same time, I knew I would not be walking off the stage with that trophy. With Cheryl by my side, I made good on my personal promise to let everybody in the room know what a treasure she was.

"As for this," I said, gesturing toward the Emmy, "there's only one place it belongs—and that's on the mantel at Stuart Scott's house. So if the girls could come up, please . . . this is not for me."

Stuart and I had worked thousands of miles apart for different networks but had crossed paths from time to time, and we had encouraged each other in our respective cancer fights over the years. I had never met his daughters, Taelor and Sydni, but I knew from experience the toll that cancer takes on a family. My own kids had struggled knowing their dad was in the fight of his life. Tae and Syd had lost their dad. They needed a blackberry moment.

And you know what's crazy? A few months later the St. Louis Sports Commission, which annually holds the Stan Musial Sportsmanship Awards, notified me that I would be receiving one of those. They wanted to give me a statue for giving one up. And that became a blackberry moment for me. Because who had they secretly arranged to be there in St. Louis to present it? Taelor and Sydni Scott.

I got a call from Roger Thompson the other day. I know what you're thinking. "Hold on . . . wait a second—*that* Roger Thompson? C'mon, you know *him*?" Actually, you're doing none of that. You've probably never heard of Roger, but if you ever did get a chance to sit and talk with him, get to know him a little, there is no doubt you'd come away proudly saying, "Yeah, I know *that* Roger Thompson."

In 1967, he was the coach of the Big Apple Tigers, a Little League Baseball team comprised of ten-, eleven-, and twelve-year-olds. Big Apple was the grocery store that sponsored the team. Tigers was the name Roger picked for us, not for some deep motivational reason but because tigers were his favorite animal. I was the ten-year-old second baseman on that team and oddly enough went by the name Tiger. It's something my dad and mom called me early on, and it actually stuck until I was about twelve. I bring that up because when Roger, who's eighty-seven now, left a message on my phone recently, just calling to touch base, he ended it by saying, "Keep up the good work, Tiger." Nobody has called me that in more than forty years.

Coach had remained good friends with my mom and dad long after I played for him, and they had passed his number on to me one day, and I'm so glad they did. Every now and then I call him or he calls me, and we talk for a minute or two, which usually becomes five or ten or thirty-seven, as it did today. I'm always amazed at his recall of exact games and situations.

I told him I'll never forget the three-word mantra he hammered home at each practice and each game of what was a championship season, the same three words that were etched on the ink pens he gave each of us at our end-of-the-season party: dedication, pride, togetherness.

We can talk about common ground now that we've both got kids out in the real world and we're both grandfathers, but in a very special way, every time I have Roger on the phone, it's like I'm having a conversation with my dad, who died at the age Coach is now. Every time we're about to hang up, he says he's proud of me, and while he's speaking to me from his home in the mountains of North Carolina, it's as if my dad were standing right there.

All of us who have put in a sufficient number of years in the parents club know that when a child becomes a teenager, the dynamic between that child and the parent can change just a bit. It can become strained just a bit. It can become difficult to some extent. It can totally implode one day, return to normalcy in the span of twenty-four hours, and then implode again with even greater force twenty minutes after that. Look, I try to be as positive, as optimistic a dad as I can possibly be. And I've always wanted my kids to know, especially during their teens, that I have the utmost confidence in them to do the right thing and make the proper decision at the proper time. Part of that comes from believing I've done the best job of parenting I could possibly do. But I've fallen short more times than I care to count.

Picture this. It happened in 1991 while Cheryl was in Romania adopting Michael. Eric is seven and Maggie is four. They're in the backseat as I pull into a parking spot right up front at the mall, thirty yards from the Macy's door. I tell them I need to run in and pick up a pair of pants that have been altered—it'll take three minutes. I tell Eric he is in charge. "Just sit tight, and I'll be back in a second." I dash inside and tell the cashier what I am there for, and he goes to a back room to get my pants. Then I see three women crouching down near the door I just entered.

"Oh, honey, don't cry. It's okay. Are your parents in this store?"

"How did you get here, sweetie? Look around. Do you see your daddy?"

Maggie had left the car and walked alone from the parking lot to the Macy's men's department, and now I am making the walk of shame to scoop her up and dry her tears, all the while being absolutely pierced by the daggers coming from the eyes of these moms. I deserve it. I was careless and stupid, and well, you probably have a few more fitting adjectives. I walk back to the car with my pants and my distraught four-year-old and of course immediately blame it all on the seven-year-old in the backseat.

"Eric, what did I tell you? You were supposed to watch your sister! What were you thinking letting her get out of the car?"

Now I have two kids bawling in the backseat, and I sit behind the wheel angry and humiliated. Not a word is spoken on the drive home. As soon as we hit the garage, the kids scramble out of the car, through the back door, and into their rooms. I sit alone at the kitchen table replaying the worst parenting episode I had yet authored. And it hits me. The parent isn't always right. The parent may make the rules, and the parent may enforce the punishment, but the parent isn't always right. While we spend a lot of time instructing our kids how to say, "I'm sorry," there are times we need a refresher course.

I call the kids downstairs, and they have a seat in the piano room, which is occasionally used for piano playing but more often is used as the place where Dad has a "come to Jesus" meeting with a child who has broken the rules. They are probably expecting a continuation of my parking lot tantrum. That's not what they get.

"Eric and Maggie, listen to me. I need to apologize to you."

Their gazes go from the carpet to my face, hitting me right between the eyes.

"What happened today at the mall wasn't your fault. It was mine. I was wrong. And I was wrong to blame you. I'm so sorry. What happened today would never have happened if I was a better parent, and I can promise you it will never happen again."

The mood in the room, as you might guess, lightens considerably. The kids hug me and forgive me as only a seven-year-old and a four-year-old can—with a simple, "That's okay, Dad." And then they go skipping out of the piano room, fully aware that on this night a request for pizza and a hot fudge sundae will not be denied. And me—well, I am thankful for a couple things. Number one, that my bone-headed move at the mall didn't result in something much worse. And number two, that I have a few more weeks before I have to explain the whole thing to Cheryl when she gets home from Romania. I'll have to have a seat in the piano room when that happens.

The lesson for me was simple. Your focus can be so razor sharp on what your kids are doing and what decisions they're making that you forget to look in the mirror sometimes and take a good, long, maybe difficult look at how you're doing. There are times when you need to step out from behind the protective shield that reads, "I'm the dad—I'm right" and admit that you made a mistake. I want my kids to have that same honesty as they're growing up and that same willingness to face up to their mistakes. Look, you may have worked your tail off to raise them the right way and to instill the values they'll need for a lifetime. Your kids have a solid foundation; they're grounded; they're "good kids" who other parents tell you are just "so polite and well mannered." But I know this. And excuse me if I offend you because I don't know what's going on under *your* roof and I haven't met *your* perfect son or daughter. And if such an animal truly exists and he or she is yours, you have my heartfelt apology. But they're gonna screw up. It's gonna happen. And it's gonna rock you.

Wayne Watson wrote a song almost twenty years ago called "Come Home," and a line in there doesn't just speak to me but screams at me in describing what it's like to be a parent and to wait up to see my kid's headlights hit the driveway so I can go to sleep: "You pray to keep from worrying, then you worry you ain't prayin' enough." Been there. How about you? I know what it's like to have a 2:35 a.m. conversation with a police officer about my child's conduct. I am familiar with the term *bail*. I am not tossing anybody under the Greyhound here. Just realize that I've been there and know what it's like to feel as though I have somehow failed as a parent.

Only by God's grace have those lapses in judgment, or downright stupid decisions, not led to something catastrophic. Certainly, there are parents out there who could write a far different story. One of heartbreak and loss. Cheryl and I are lucky. The kids are all still around, living their lives, making us proud, making us cringe, and on a regular basis providing us with blackberries.

It didn't take long after we adopted Carmen from Paraguay for Cheryl and me to realize that she was going to do things at her pace. When she was just four years old, her room was routinely a disaster area. One morning we offered her a dollar if she would clean her room. She was thrilled and ran upstairs while Cheryl and I high-fived. Ten minutes later she came back downstairs and said, "Thanks anyway" and gave Cheryl the dollar back. She would eventually get it done, but doing it when we requested apparently wasn't worth the princely sum we had offered her.

When Carmen was fifteen, she would ride to church with me and Cheryl and Michael and then would vanish. Our church, 12 Stone, features a circular auditorium that seats twenty-six hundred. Carmen and her high school friends would sit as far away from us as possible and still be within the confines of the church. One particular Sunday Pastor Kevin Myers, in the midst of his message, felt moved to offer to anyone in the church a chance to be baptized—right then. We hadn't pressured Carmen on this in the past. We had had discussions about it and had pointed out that most of her friends had been baptized, but we didn't want her to do it because it was *our* wish but because she had reached a point in her spiritual growth where it was what *she* wanted. And apparently, this was that day. Cheryl elbowed me and pointed toward the stage, where among the first to step forward was our Carmen.

An unscripted moment like that can't be put on the calendar in advance. It can't be the work of a mom and dad double-team breaking down a teenager's resolve. That was just a moment between Carmen and the God who made her. And we got to see it.

Our family of six became a family of eight after my wife and I had both hit our fifties. While some of our friends were figuring out the cool ways they could spend their new free time with no kids in the house, we were not. While we had known for a long time that the empty nester thing wasn't going to happen in our house, with Michael needing constant care, that didn't mean we had to add two more kids to the mix, but that's what happened. The initial suggestion to adopt again came from Cheryl, who while leading the Street Grace fight against child sex trafficking had told me that many of the young women who age out of the foster care system get caught in the sex trade. They are targets for pimps, who give them the attention, or money, or personal value they so desperately crave but then in no time have them under their control. Some of these young women are performing dozens of sex acts in a single day—every day.

When Cheryl brought up the idea of adopting a girl out of foster care, a girl who might fall into the trap I detailed above, I did not jump on board immediately. Not that I didn't see the need. I just thought the adoption ship not only had sailed but also was circling the globe and would never stop by our port again. But the more Cheryl and I talked, the more adoption became not something we *could* do but something we *should* do.

We wouldn't be adopting an infant but an older child who was about to enter a very formative period of her life. So we made ourselves available. That has kind of an Old Testament feel to it, like the prophet Isaiah answering the Lord's "Whom shall I send?" with a "Here I am, send me." Turns out we didn't adopt a girl. We adopted two. Ashley, nine, and Allison, ten, were half sisters (same mom, different dads). They had bounced around half a dozen foster homes. There had been abuse in their past. They had learning disabilities. I would tell my friends that the girls didn't have many possessions, but they had a lot of baggage. Unpacking it was difficult. We were trying to show them love. They were trying to trust that we were not going to be just another stop on the road. Early on there was this unforgettable exchange between Cheryl and Allison that spoke to the heart of the struggle.

"Allison, you have to realize that this is it. This is your forever home."

"I have a question."

"Go ahead, hon."

"How long will forever be this time?"

I would love to spin a tale of how Allison and Ashley walked into their new home and were so overcome with gratitude, so thrilled with this new "forever" opportunity that their past quickly faded from memory and we all lived happily ever after. That would be a lie. It was so hard. I'll be brutally honest here. Cheryl and I wondered if we had done the right thing, if we had overestimated our ability to parent a couple girls who had endured *their* life experience.

At times, the two of us had controlled, commonsense, matter-of-fact conversations about it. On one of those occasions, we were strolling through a sprawling local park and got so wrapped up in the discussion that we took a wrong turn and got . . . lost. It was a fitting metaphor for where we were mentally in that early stage after the adoption. After finding our way to a parking lot, we actually had to beg a ride from a woman who was backing out of a parking spot, and she drove us three miles to where we had left our car. Sometimes those conversations got heated, and we hated what those differences of opinion were doing to us as a couple. I was in Orlando one night when Cheryl called to tell me about the most recent incident of unacceptable behavior by one of the girls, and I was furious.

"So is this what you wanted, Cheryl? Is this really what you wanted?"

"This isn't what either of us wanted, but I didn't think this was about what we *wanted* but what we felt *called* to do."

She was right. And that was a defining moment for us. We rediscovered our purpose in bringing these two young girls into our family. Rather than expending so much energy sparring over who had the better idea about how to raise them and how they were affecting us, we determined to simply focus on the girls and what would be best for their future, understanding and accepting that it would not be easy.

Allison and Ashley are in their teens now, and we still unpack their baggage from time to time. The truth is some of my bags have turned up too. The one labeled "patience" is pretty heavy. I had to pick the lock on the one called "understanding" so I could remember the background of these new Johnson girls. And I couldn't quite remember the combination to that designer piece called "joy" until I realized that circumstances, difficulties, and roadblocks can't steal joy. Turns out that bag wasn't even locked—I just didn't know how to open it. But I'm continuing to learn in a process that's had blackberries *and* thorns. If it's all right with you, I'll just keep my focus on the blackberries.

I've never been a big car guy. I can drive 'em and wash 'em, and that's about it. If somebody tells me about a '63 "this" with a "whatever" engine, I don't even know enough about it to be impressed. And forget about car repair of any type. Look, I've changed a few tires through the years and always proudly walked around the house with my grime-covered shirt, just hoping somebody would ask about it. "Oh, this? Yeah . . . I uh . . changed a tire on the van today. It was pretty tough. Those lug nuts were on there pretty good. But I got it done—myself. Phew, that tire changing . . . that's no joke."

Well, when you have a son like Michael, who has this Rain Man–type fixation with and memory about cars, you find yourself at the auto show in downtown Atlanta every year. I'm still not a car guy, but I've seen every new model for the last fifteen years in the course of a four-hour trip through the Georgia World Congress Center with Michael. That show is like a Christmas in April blackberry for him.

My buddy Phil Bollier, Michael's high school basketball coach, obviously knows about his fascination with cars and for his eighteenth birthday thought it would be cool for him

201

to take a ride in a convertible. So Phil arranged with a Ford dealership to borrow a Mustang for the afternoon. It took a little finagling with a portable lift system, but I was able to lower Michael into the front seat and strap him in. Maggie sat in the backseat shooting video, and we drove around for a half hour. This was a treat for Michael, who always rides in a van sitting in his wheelchair.

We came home, cut the cake, and popped the video in. You could hear the roar of the engine, see the wind whipping through Michael's hair, and not help but see the huge smile on his face as he experienced something he hadn't done since becoming wheelchair-bound six years earlier.

The story doesn't end there. Cheryl is the financial wizard of our house. She has always known, down to the penny, our balance. The video of Michael in that convertible was pretty powerful. Cheryl bought that used Mustang, and here's how she explained it: "There's no way in the world I was going to see you guys share a moment like that just once. Ernie, we're lucky, we're blessed, we can afford it. I just had to do it."

We've had that Mustang for ten years now, and every time I take it in for service, the technician is amazed at how few miles are on the odometer, and I tell him I drive it only on special occasions. Those are spring or fall days when the temperature is just right—when the sun won't bake us or the wind won't make us shiver. Even now with the ventilator Michael's constant companion and the extra gear we need to bring along, I can still lower Michael into the passenger seat. I can still make him toss his head back and laugh when I fire up the engine. We'll drive around for a few hours, play our music loud and sing off-key, and maybe swing by a friend's house. It's not the destination; it's the journey.

And those trips—well, just call me the driver who's along for the ride.

———— ◦ ————

I love Sunday dinner. It doesn't matter what we're having; it's all about who we're having over. For years, it's been this way. It really started to become a "thing" when I discovered that my father-in-law, Lou Deluca, could fix anything. I don't mean "fix" as in preparing dinner. I mean, he could fix whatever was broken in our house, and he has always been more than happy to display his skills while at the same time chuckling at my inability to master anything in the household repair realm. Oftentimes, he and my mother-in-law, Joan, would come over, and Lou would fix the vacuum, or repair a leaky faucet, or fix a toilet that wouldn't stop running, and Cheryl and I would talk them into staying for dinner. Now it's a Sunday night Johnson tradition, and Lou isn't required to bring his toolbox.

When I was growing up in Milwaukee and later Atlanta, I rarely saw my grandparents. Thorwald and Inkie lived in Vermont, and Nenny and Koko were in California, so the opportunities were rare. I love the fact that my kids see their grandparents all the time, and Sunday dinner has become the perfect vehicle for nurturing that relationship and for reminding all of us that when you get right down to it, there's nothing quite like family.

Aside from figuring out what we'll cook, and it can range from burgers, to barbecued chicken, to Cheryl's world-famous lasagna, there's really no big plan that goes into those Sunday nights. No theme, no dress code, no script. There might be a ball game on TV, Lou might be watching an old Western, Cheryl and Joan might be comparing notes on what their vegetable gardens are producing, or we might be gathered around the fireplace on the back patio on a cool fall evening.

The kids and their spouses and their kids come over. It's a four-generation celebration. Depending on how you read the calendar, it's the greatest way either to end or to start the week. It's always a tangible recognition of how blessed we are to have that group gathered around that table on that night, with every dinner preceded by a shared blessing. One at a time we take a moment to say what we're thankful for, and we close with the refrain "Because God is good all the time, and all the time, God is good." And oh yeah, there's Michael's period on that sentence: "Amen. Eat now."

Sometimes blackberries come when there is nobody around. They come in what seem to be those all-too-rare moments of solitude when you're able to wander at least fifteen feet away from your phone without suffering text withdrawal. That probably isn't an *actual* condition, but it wouldn't surprise me if one of these nights we hear on the 6:00 news that it indeed is. And then, of course, there will be a drug for it and a sixty-second commercial used to sell it, with a frightening list of side effects that range from hair loss to unsightly rashes to night terrors. And, of course, there will be a warning that if you feel a need to read emails for four hours, see a doctor.

For me, that place of solitude can be as close as the back-yard or as remote as a deserted beach at sunrise. In those moments, it's just me and my camera. We have half a dozen bird feeders scattered around the backyard, a couple of those for hummingbirds, and there are birdhouses where every year we can watch wrens and eastern bluebirds build their nests and have their babies, and we've watched those young'uns try out their wings for the first time. I've taken thousands of pictures of baby birds screaming their heads off, craning their necks to get some food from Mom. I've captured that brilliant, indescribable shade of blue that marks the eastern bluebird and the vivid yellow of the goldfinch.

I've also sat patiently a few yards from a feeder filled with sugar water just waiting for a hummingbird to flash into view, hover for a second or two, and then vanish as quickly as it appeared. If you've ever been close enough not just to see but also to *hear* a hummingbird in flight, you know it's pretty amazing. In times like that, I always find myself marveling at creation, and when I start going down that path, I'm often overcome with a deep feeling of gratitude. Granted, my family and I are a very small and very ordinary part of this huge, sprawling, limitless, and extraordinary creation, but hey, we're a part of it! And membership brings the opportunity to sit and soak and rest in the knowledge that I've been blessed beyond recognition.

Speaking of being blessed, you know what I'll always remember about the Hawaiian island of Kauai? They used to play the PGA Grand Slam of Golf there, and the company actually paid me to go and call the action. Two days of work in a weeklong stay. Grueling. From year to year, the season's four major champions would make the trip and play thirty-six holes. So the likes of Tiger Woods, Phil Mickelson, Davis Love III, and Ernie Els were regulars. That in itself made the event special, but what I'll never forget is the sunrise.

There's a cliff that juts out into Poipu Bay on Kauai. During the day, the more adventurous vacationers jump from it and make the long swim to shore. But I loved to visit that cliff before the sun came up. Again, just me and my camera. I would change lenses and angles as the sun slowly and elegantly made its daily appearance, and I swear I was looking at shades and hues that I don't think actually have names. It was breathtaking, and it ushered me into that nebulous and wonderful space of gratitude again, where all I could manage was an "Alleluia."

The show went on. I made the trek back down from the cliff to the beach and heard something I'd never heard before. As the tide leisurely made its way to shore, it washed over thousands of small rocks (nearly the size of a golf ball, I'd say). They were black or charcoal gray, not uniform in any way, with indentations and holes of various shapes. As the waters receded, these rocks moved in unison ever so slightly, clicking against each other, creating the most unique sound—low, rumbling, rich, and almost hypnotic. I later learned from a local that these were lava rocks and that perhaps one of the reasons for the unique sound was that some were more hollowed out than others. For a half hour I sat there mesmerized by this unscripted symphony. I still have one of those lava rocks sitting on my dresser as a reminder of that day, that sound, that Creator.

In April 2015, I was asked to speak at the YMCA of Atlanta Good Friday breakfast, a nondenominational event that had been held every year for the last fifty. I was invited to tell my "faith story" to a room of several hundred people.

My schedule was tight that day. I needed to leave afterward and get to the airport for a flight to Indianapolis and the NCAA Final Four.

I called my speech "The Unscripted Life" and used a series of photographs: the Little League team where the original blackberry story took root, me and my dad, Cheryl in the Romanian orphanage with Michael, me hairless after chemo, Michael on Phil Bollier's basketball team, a group shot of our six kids. I talked about "trusting God . . . period" and living in awe of how God orchestrates life and connects the dots in remarkable ways. And I told them about the marvelous gift Cheryl gave me one December day several years earlier. To mark my spiritual birthday one year, she gave me a compass, which was beautiful. But what made it so special was the handwritten note attached to it that simply said, "Remembering the day you found your direction." I've told that story many times to many groups, and the moment when I show the compass and talk about that note—well, it's always hard to get through, because the gesture just meant so much.

As the audience was dismissed, some hustled off to work, others stayed and mingled, and still others came toward my table. I had about thirty minutes before I needed to leave for the airport and spent that time meeting folks, taking pictures, and signing programs. I heard stories similar to mine from cancer survivors and adoptive parents, and I checked my watch to make sure I was still on schedule.

When I looked up, the man in front of me asked if I recognized him. I told him he'd have to help me, and he identified himself. For the purposes of this story, I'm just going to call him MD. When he said his name, I felt sick. We had not seen each other since seventh or eighth grade—about forty-five years. I had bullied MD back then—made fun of him, tried to goad him into a fight that he wanted no part of, and then punched him anyway. When I became a parent and lectured my kids about treating classmates the right way and never being the bully, I always knew I was a world-class hypocrite because of what I had done to MD. For years, it stuck in my mind, but I'd try to rationalize it with the age-old "boys will be boys" argument.

And now here he stood.

As we made small talk about our families and our jobs and where we lived, I felt an intense prompting to bring up that painful story from the past and to say I was sorry.

And I fought it off.

I tried to convince myself that MD probably didn't even remember it, so there was no reason to go there, but as we were shaking hands and about to end this unscripted meeting, I couldn't fight it any longer.

"MD, I need to be as absolutely transparent here as I can. A long time ago I treated you the wrong way. I was a bully, and it's bothered me ever since. I don't even know if you remember, but I had to say it."

"Ernie, I was hoping you had forgotten."

"No chance. So all I can do at this point, forty-five years later, is say I'm sorry and to ask if after all this time you can forgive me."

"It's done."

It was the most amazing snapshot of God's grace I could possibly imagine. There were still people waiting to speak with me, but now they stood watching these two men who hadn't seen each other in ages hugging, tears in their eyes. On a day when I had told people to be on the lookout for blackberry moments, those times when you're blown away by how God orchestrates life, here I was being absolutely floored by that very thing.

Can I leave you with something that I hope doesn't sound too simplistic? I am fully aware that it probably will, but here goes.

I love this life.

It's easy for me to say that when I consider I grew up with loving parents who were married longer than I've been alive and I have a beautiful wife of thirty-four years, great kids, a granddaughter, Katie, and a grandson, Ernest Everett, who love to be held by their grandfather, whom they call Poppy, which is what their parents called their grandfather. And hey, there are millions of guys out there who would trade jobs with me in a heartbeat. I mean, what's not to love?

Nothing.

That includes facing every day the fact that Michael has a fatal disease, enduring those times when the thought of cancer coming back barges into my mind, having a question that only my dad can answer but having no way to ask him, and feeling like I've lost my touch as a parent because my words aren't getting through and my patience is running on E.

Yep, even in those times when it's depressing, scary, or frustrating, I wouldn't change a thing.

Really.

I may be naïve but not naïve enough to believe in such a thing as a trouble-free life. We all have "stuff" to deal with, and the stuff our family has is different from the stuff yours has. And so your stories are going to have different twists and turns, and you're going to have moments on mountaintops, and you're going to spend what seems like an eternity in the valley. But for the most part, you're going to be doing life somewhere in the middle, where if you're not overly preoccupied with the goal of simply making it from this day to the next, you might notice for the first time blackberries ripe for the picking.

And you may notice that love and loss and hope and desperation and courage and understanding and sorrow and exhilaration and forgiveness all live there. And you may just find that they all seem to make more sense when you trust God . . . period.

Yeah, I love this life.

And living it unscripted.

ACKNOWLEDGMENTS

THIS IS THE PART of the book where I thank everybody. Now if it were one of those televised awards shows, I'm sure the "Hey, you're out of time, get off the stage" music would begin playing, and I would have to rush through the last few names and hope I didn't leave anybody out. That's one of the beauties of the printed page. I can take my time. But I'm still worried I'll leave someone out.

Since I'd never written a book, I needed a literary agent who could walk me through every step of this totally foreign landscape. A handful of intrepid souls offered to take that on. I couldn't have made a better decision than choosing to work with Chris Park. She's an amazing woman whose patience, honesty, and encouragement carried me through the entire process. And it still brings a smile to my face when she refers to me as "one of her authors." Unreal.

When it came time to select a publisher for *Unscripted*, again I had choices, and I am so grateful to those who wanted to be a part of helping me tell this story. But there was something special about Baker Publishing Group. I'll never forget the long-distance video conference we had in the spring of 2016 when editorial director Chad Allen, executive vice president of trade publishing Jennifer Leep, marketing manager Eileen Hanson, and sales director Nate Henrion laid out for me Baker's plans for the book. We were thousands of miles apart physically that morning, but it felt like we were gathered around the kitchen table. It's an honor to be a part of the Baker family and to have brothers and sisters like Mark Rice, Brianna DeWitt, Brian Vos, Kristin Kornoelje, Michelle Bardin, Patti Brinks, and Erin Bartels.

Thanks to my lifelong representatives at Career Sports and Entertainment (CSE): Lonnie Cooper, Mark Carmony, Mark Burns, Bobby Height, Amy Lowe, David Koonan, and Molly Fletcher. Your guidance and friendship can't be measured.

Since 1989, I have had a home at Turner Broadcasting and have worked with some of the most influential figures in television. David Levy stands at the top of the list. There couldn't be a better boss or a finer man. I'm indebted to Don McGuire and the late Robert Wussler for believing in me way back when and signing me to that first Turner contract. In the twenty-eight years that followed, I've had the distinct pleasure of working for Mark Lazarus, Mike Pearl, Harvey Schiller, Ned Simon, and Jeff Behnke. These days I am privileged to work under the leadership of Lenny Daniels, Craig Barry, Tara August, Albert "Scooter" Vertino, and Tim Kiely. What a group. I can't forget the folks who get me from assignment to assignment and city to city—Michelle Zarzaca, Ben Spitalnick, and Olivia Scarlett—and, of course, our Turner public relations team headed up by Sal Petruzzi in New York and Nate Smeltz in Atlanta.

Thanks to Charles Barkley, Kenny Smith, and Shaquille O'Neal for being the brothers I never had, and to Ron Darling, Cal Ripken Jr., John Smoltz, Dennis Eckersley, David Wells, Buck Martinez, and Joe Simpson for being such tremendous partners in the broadcast booth, where I feel blessed to sit and do what my father did for so many years—call baseball games. Thanks to my pals in the eighteenth tower at the PGA Championship and British Open: Bill Kratzert, Ian Baker Finch, Bobby Clampett, Paul Azinger, Jim Nantz, and Mike Tirico—true friends and professionals. And I can't forget the late Jim Huber—there's never been a better writer in television or a better dinner companion on the road. As for Craig Sager, I'm at a loss to adequately describe how I've valued his friendship, the joy he's always gotten from going to work, and his absolutely remarkable public battle with leukemia that has inspired people worldwide.

And, of course, there's another group to recognize. My family. I can't say much more about them than what you've already read. When somebody asks me how long Cheryl and I have been married, my answer is, "Not long enough." For the record, it will be thirty-five years this summer. To this day, I have no idea how I got so lucky. To my kids, Eric, Maggie, Michael, Carmen, Allison, and Ashley—I am honored to be your dad, and there are no words to describe how proud you make me every day. To Dustin Pruitt and Quynh Truong—you're the greatest son-in-law and daughter-in-law that a father-in-law could ever hope for. To Lou and Joan Deluca—I don't know why so many people joke about their in-laws. You two are an absolute treasure. And you raised an amazing daughter.

Thanks to my mom, Lois, as inspiring and loving a person as has ever walked this planet. Thanks to my sisters, Dawn and Chris, who did what all big sisters do to their baby brothers—protected, encouraged, terrorized, and above all, loved him with all their hearts. And, Chris, thanks for organizing the annual March Madness bracket, which magically brings us all together in the midst of our busyness. It's always very humbling to see my name trailing the likes of you and Dawn; and our niece, Rebecca; and Mom; and Cheryl; and the list goes on and on.

And finally, to Katie Ann Pruitt and Ernest Everett Johnson. You're a little young right now, but one day you'll read this book written by your grandfather Poppy. When that day comes, I hope you'll see that you're the two newest members of a family built on the foundation of unconditional love . . . and nourished by blackberries. You just can't script that.

Notes

1. John Lombardo and John Ourand, "Fast Break—NBA Media Rights," *Sports Business Daily/Sports Business Journal*, December 11, 2014.

2. John Ortberg, *Soul Keeping: Caring for the Most Important Part of You* (Grand Rapids: Zondervan, 2014).

3. "Little Miss Magic" (Jimmy Buffet) © 1981 Coral Reefer Music (BMI). ALL RIGHTS RESERVED. USED BY PERMISSION.

Ernie Johnson Jr. is a three-time Sports Emmy Award winner and host of TNT's *Inside the NBA* with Charles Barkley, Kenny Smith, and Shaquille O'Neal. He is the studio host for NBA TV's popular *Fan Night* and a studio host for Turner and CBS's NCAA Division I Men's Basketball Championship coverage. He is the lead play-by-play announcer for Turner's coverage of Major League Baseball and the PGA Championship, and has also covered the National Football League, The British Open, Wimbledon, and the Olympics. In 2007, Johnson was presented with the first-ever honorary John Wooden Keys to Life Award, presented by Athletes in Action, which is awarded to individuals who exemplify Wooden's "Seven Keys to Life," including character, integrity, and faith. In 2015, he was recognized with a Musial Award, presented in honor of Stan Musial's legacy by celebrating iconic "good sports" and the year's greatest moments in sportsmanship. In 2016, his alma mater, the University of Georgia, honored him with the Grady College of Journalism John Holliman Lifetime Achievement Award as well as the Bill Hartman Award for Lifetime Achievement from the UGA Athletic Department. Johnson lives in Braselton, Georgia, with his wife, Cheryl, and their six children, four of whom are adopted.

Connect with *Ernie*!

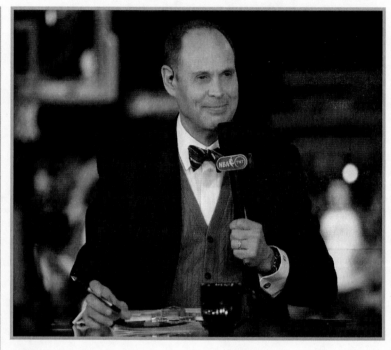

 @TurnerSportsEJ | @Ernie.Johnson

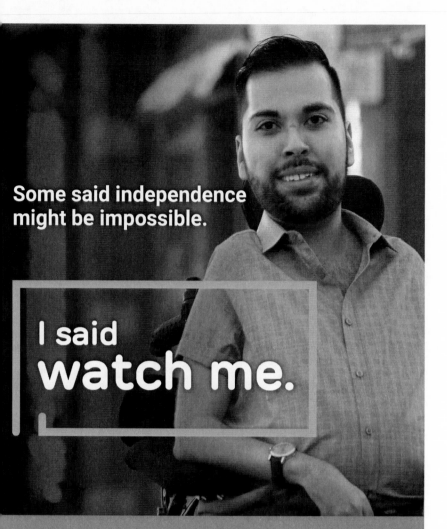

Some said independence might be impossible.

I said
watch me.

"My doctors told me I wouldn't live past 12 years old. They told my parents I wouldn't go to high school or graduate from college. I'm grateful to have proven them wrong."
– Joe Akmakjian, living with spinal muscular atrophy

Help more individuals like Joe live longer and grow stronger by donating to the Muscular Dystrophy Association today at mda.org. Your support will give strength, independence, and life through groundbreaking research, care, and support.

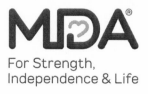

MDA®
For Strength,
Independence & Life

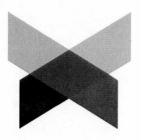
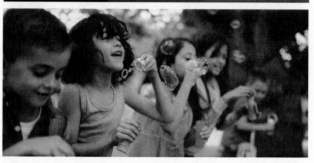
 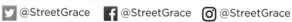

Made in United States
North Haven, CT
23 May 2022